WITHIN LIFE'S SPAN

12 MSC   S40019

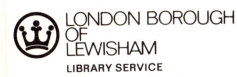

WITHIN LIFE'S SPAN

PROFESSOR ROBERT HUGHES PARRY

M.D.(Lond.), F.R.C.P.(Lond.), D.P.H.
formerly Honorary Physician to H.M. King George VI
and to H.M. Queen Elizabeth II

ARTHUR H. STOCKWELL LTD.
Elms Court   Ilfracombe
Devon

© *R. Hughes Parry, 1973*
First published in Great Britain, 1973

SBN 7223 0537-0
PRINTED IN GREAT BRITAIN BY
ARTHUR H. STOCKWELL LTD.
Elms Court   -   Ilfracombe
Devon

ACKNOWLEDGEMENTS

I am very grateful to Sir Thomas Parry Williams for his assistance. Not only did he read the MSS. and make valuable comments but he also translated into English, for the purpose of this book, original Welsh verses by himself and others.

To my good friends of school days and later I give my best thanks for allowing me to draw freely from their photo albums and to reproduce the pictures which I hope they will enjoy in the book.

Finally without the help of Joan this book would not have been written; it is indeed a joint effort.

*To our Grandchildren, with love and best wishes
from Taid and Nain.
May you have pleasure and encouragement
from the story of our life's span*

CONTENTS

*"Under the Cherry Tree" published 1969
Gomerian Press

LIST OF ILLUSTRATIONS

FOREWORD

This is a study of a small rural community in South Caernarfonshire since the beginning of the century. Having known the author since his young days, I know too of his great love for this part of Wales and his deep interest in all that concerns it.

The book tells of the changes that have occurred in the appearance of the countryside as well as in the life of the district.

Doctor Hughes Parry had the advantage of returning to his native heath when he came back to practise as a family doctor not many miles from his birthplace. At the time of writing he is living in retirement in the same area, and can appreciate the further changes that have taken place in the last forty years.

It is only natural that a doctor should pay special attention to family and home life, especially from a social and medical viewpoint. Comparison of home doctoring of yesterday and today has been made in the light of the National Health and modern Social Services.

It is with much pleasure that I commend WITHIN LIFE'S SPAN which records so faithfully and sympathetically the impressions of one who is specially qualified to review the changing scene.

T. H. Parry Williams

Aberystwyth.

I. THE TURN OF THE CENTURY

"O! Gwyn fy myd pan oeddwn gynt
Yn llanc di-boen ar lwybrau'r gwynt."

Cynan

O! blest was I in bygone days
A carefree lad on windy ways.
English translation by Sir Thomas Parry Williams.

Our Village

Jutting out into the Irish Sea is the part of South Caernarfonshire known as the Llŷn Peninsula. Away to the north east of this peninsula lie Yr Eifl (the Rivals), a range of mountains at the foot of whose southern slopes lies the village of Llanhaelhaearn. This little village and its surroundings with its people and their activities are portrayed as I remember them at the beginning of this century.

My home was a farm called Uwchlaw'rffynnon (Above the Well) about half a mile up the hillside from the centre of the village.

Llanhaelhaearn was, and still is, a compact little village of stone houses and buildings either side of a

narrow street leading down to the main road from
Pwllheli to Caernarfon, and spreading for a short
distance along this road. The village is surrounded
on all sides by hills, except for two gaps, a narrow
one to the north through which one catches a glimpse
of the Menai Straits and Anglesey, and the other to
the south, giving a panorama of the countryside as
far as the sea and the coast of Cardiganshire. Above
the village, on either side of the valley, houses give
way to small fields bounded by stone walls with, here
and there, a farmhouse and its buildings breaking up
the patchwork pattern. To the north of the village the
small green fields are overshadowed by the rocky peak
of Tre'Ceiri and the range of Yr Eifl. These slopes
with hardly a tree to be seen, are bright with the
colour of heather and gorse growing between the stony
outcrops in the summer time. At other times they are
shrouded in mist and rain, or on wintry days may be
covered with snow, but the effect of the nearness of
the sea and the southerly aspect provides a less
rigorous climate than in many other parts of the
country. When occasionally the north wind blows, its
icy blast can be felt through the gap in the hills to the
north. On the other hand the full force of the south
westerly gales comes across the Peninsula from
Cardigan Bay, and many a night I can remember
listening to it howling through the few trees outside
my bedroom window.

There were legends associated with the hills and
mountains, and interest in their history was stimulated
by Baring Gould when he stayed at our house in 1903.
I was only about seven years old at the time but his
discoveries were exciting to young and old. He was
carrying out excavations on the summit of Tre'Ceiri
to find the armed camps that had been built by the
Irish after the Romans had left, and the Irish had
tried to seize control of the Llŷn Peninsula. The
remains of a fort can now be seen enclosing the 'huts

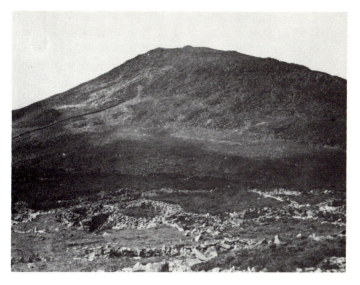

Cytiau'r gwyddelod (Irish huts)

of the Irish', (Cytiau'r gwyddelod) if one climbs to the top of the mountain. Because of its comparative inaccessibility there has been very little damage to these archaeological remains by visitors.

The village had a population of about two hundred and fifty. The houses were small and built of stone with roofs of slate from near-by quarries. There was an old Church and graveyard at the top of the narrow street overlooking the village. Lower down were the school and a small Chapel. Another Chapel could be seen some distance along a road into the hills to the west. There was no village green or playing field and the children had to be content with a school yard, which could only be used during school hours. But with the hills and fields in which to roam, the need for more space was not so important in those days.

There were only three small shops selling everything from bread and paraffin to ropes and nails, and two small sweet shops where one could buy a halfpenny-worth of liquorice in a long string, pepperminty sweets and sticks of candy that I have not seen for many years.

The water supply for the villagers may not have been convenient but there was never a shortage from the wells and springs in the area. There was no piped water to the houses but in two or three places in the village there were taps for water piped from a well on the hillside. Most of the farms had their own supply from a well or spring, and the streams coming down the mountains meant additional water for the animals.

Naturally there was no indoor plumbing or sanitation in the houses, but there were always plenty of tin basins and an extra large one for a good scrub on Saturday nights! There was a privy midden in the garden and commodes were often used in emergencies or cases of sickness.

In olden times the village well was supposed to be a holy well and the bubbling of the water (from the spring underneath!) was looked upon as 'the troubling of the waters' and was said to have had miraculous power to heal. Often sick persons would come to drink the water and even to bathe in it to try and effect a cure. In our days this old well used to have a low stone wall protecting it, with stone seats around, but it was easily accessible from the road. Later it was decided to erect a stone building around it as a precaution against contamination and the strong door was kept locked. As I passed this every day on my way to school I read the inscription on a slate above the door which is still there today:

Saint Aelhaern's Well
Roofed 1900.

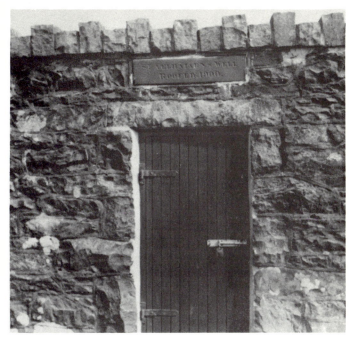

Saint Aelhaern's Well

Saint Aelhaern was the servant of Saint Beuno — and there were almost as many saints in Wales as in Ireland when he was alive. The legend associated with him was that he had acquired his name Aelhaern, meaning Iron Eyebrow, after he had been killed by wild beasts. Saint Beuno had picked up his bones, and when he noticed that part of his eyebrow was missing he fitted a piece of his own iron pikestaff in its place.

There was a sturdily built public house in the centre of the village on the main road. However, because of the influence of the chapels it did not play an important part in the lives of the villagers, nor of the farming community. It was chiefly patronised by people passing, and by men living some distance away from the village. A travelling carpenter with his donkey and cart lived about a mile away, and always succeeded in finding himself on Friday evening outside the Inn on his way home. The donkey waited patiently outside for his master. On one occasion, when the old man came out of the Inn door, he was surprised to find the donkey and cart had disappeared. He was sorely puzzled until some of the lads standing by suggested he might look in the stable. There, sure enough, was the donkey facing the doorway with the cart hitched behind it. The doorway was much too narrow to enable the cart to be driven out, and it was obvious that the cart must have been dismantled and reassembled in order to get it into the stable. The young folk standing around were apparently puzzled as to how this could have happened, but the old man's observation was much more practical. Said he "The question is not how it got in, but how to get it out."

It was not uncommon for practical jokes of this kind to be played on anyone found under the influence of drink. There was not much interference from the law in those days and the victim had learnt to expect these mischievous pranks. It was told of a well known farmer, who made a habit of drinking rather heavily at least once a week, that he never worried about getting home safely as he relied on his old pony. One evening as usual he was put in his light cart, and the pony's head set in the right direction for his home, about two miles from the public house, and started on its way. In the morning he woke up, having slept on the floor of the cart, to find his pony had disappeared. He was still dazed, and found that he was only half way home. He rubbed his eyes and said "If I am who I think I am, I have lost a pony, but if I am someone else, I have found a cart."

Apart from the traders and shopkeepers there were only two kinds of employment for the men of the district — to work on the land or in the nearby granite quarry at Trefor. In the beginning of the century the granite was in great demand and the quarry employed about a thousand men. A number of these came from our village, but most from the village of Trefor; there were also immigrant workers from other parts, some from as far away as Yorkshire. Many of them settled down and married local Welsh girls. The hours of work were long and conditions hard, but they found enjoyment in forming a brass band which became a popular entertainment in the district. We often heard them on Saturday afternoons marching up from Trefor and playing in the village street.

In the centre of the village, at the crossroads, was the village blacksmith and it was one of our greatest 'treats' as children to be allowed to go with the horses when they went to the blacksmith's to be shod. The blacksmith himself was an austere man and did not encourage children about the place.

Some Village Personalities

Opposite the Chapel and just below the Church was the cobbler's workshop, reached by a short flight of stone steps. It was a long, narrow room with a low ceiling, about seventeen feet by nine with a fair sized window facing north. It had three benches. It was fascinating to watch the cobbler at work beating and sewing and we children often wondered in those days why he never seemed to have black nails from knocking his fingers, which we did so easily. He was a short old man with a wooden leg. He had no children at home, but that did not stop him from inviting us occasionally to tea on Sundays. I never enjoyed those tea parties for the cakes were always stale and I always stuck to bread, butter and jam. In his younger days he was a good singer and conductor and often had a successful party of singers at the local Eisteddfod. However, that was before my day; but everyone enjoyed the story about Ifan the shoe-maker coming slowly up the road from his allotment with a small bucket apparently full of new potatoes and the first crop of rhubarb. The mystery of how he produced many of these good things before anyone else was exploded when one of the village lads came cycling down the street, without efficient brakes and knocked old Ifan's bucket for six, scattering its contents. The contents were revealed to be mostly rhubarb leaves, many small potatoes, a few reasonable ones and very few sticks of rhubarb!

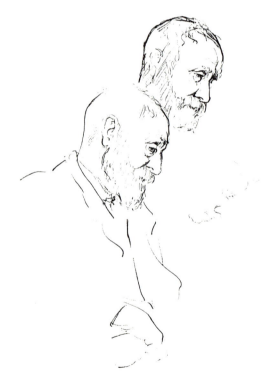

Sketch — Owen Williams

Owen Williams, who kept the Chapel House, was a tall, well built man, slightly bald; he worked as a sett maker in the granite quarry. He used to take an active part in the work of the Chapel but, to his great disappointment he was never appointed a deacon. It might have been because his brother who kept a flourishing grocer's shop in the village had already achieved this honour. On Saturday afternoons he often came up to our farm and gave a helping hand with the farm work, especially at harvest time. I mention Owen Williams because when we had moved from the village to our second home, a farm near Pwllheli, I was allowed to return to the village and stay with him and his wife Mary and their unmarried daughter. I was then about eight or nine years of age. The time was early summer but I can remember very little of what went on in the outside world. However, I did get a glimpse into the life of a quarryman in those days and the picture of his family life has stayed with me ever since.

At that time he was grey and somewhat bald and at a guess he may have been about sixty years old. His wife was a buxom little woman, quiet as a rule but could be very out-spoken when roused. They had two other children besides the rather delicate daughter who lived with them; a married son who worked on a farm away from home and a daughter married to a tradesman living in Liverpool. It was no mean achievement to bring up three children as they did, with wages as they were at that time, but as long as Owen Williams could keep working there was no great strain on the family exchequer.

I used to wake up with the dawn and although all the doors and windows were shut in the little house I could hear the old man praying fervently for about ten minutes after he had breakfasted and before leaving for the quarry. Then he went off with a pack containing his coat and overalls, a tin of sandwiches

and a tin can of tea. I could see him from my bedroom window walking up the hill joined by some fellow
workers, together they walked on up the hill past the
Chapel and the school and disappeared from sight
round the corner of the cemetery. He had a three
mile tramp to the part of the granite quarry where
his allotted "bank" was. Here he sat down on a stone
seat covered with a sack to shape the "setts". This
was the most skilled occupation in the quarry. The
trimmed stones were required for building and road
paving and were transported by steamers from the
little port of Trefor. Late in the evening he and his
mates would come home, and after washing and
changing into another suit he would sit down and enjoy
a "high tea" and a rest in his armchair by the fireplace. This was not too bad in the spring and summer
but in the winter when the mornings were dark he had
to judge the time of leaving home so that he would

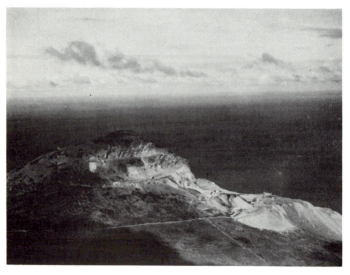

Trefor Quarry

arrive at the quarry when it would be light enough to start work. For wet weather the men had made a stone shelter that would protect them from the rain and enable them to get on with their work. The wages were small and the men were paid for what they produced so they could not afford to waste any daylight or be held up by bad weather. Mary Williams made sure there was no waste in the home and looked after Owen's clothes and her own so that they seldom had to buy new garments. But in spite of hard work and little money it was a happy home. They used to spend evenings by the fire with occasional visits from friends or a meeting in the Chapel. The minister was given board and lodging by them at the week-end for which additional expense their recompense was hardly adequate. Even at that early age I realised how important was the week-end break for the quarry workers. They could not possibly last out the whole seven days without a break. The Bible played a very important part in their lives. In fact it was the only book I saw in the house apart from a "Commentary" to help with its understanding. There were no public libraries and the few books that found their way into the village were usually passed around and these had to be in Welsh.

There was a carpenter in the village — a "bit of a wag" was the way he was usually described; he had been a ship's carpenter and had seen something of the world. It was said he was the only person ever to beat Nellie of the sweet shop at her own game. She spent most of her time chatting over the counter, commiserating with the sick and holding forth on her own illnesses. When Jacob the carpenter called round one day she started in her usual way comparing complaints. Jacob enumerated his illnesses and, sure enough, Nellie had had them all. When Jacob started telling her of his experiences with a black woman in Africa Nellie threw up her hands in dismay and exclaimed "Oh no, I never had anything like that."

There was a policeman in the village, but it was a well behaved community and he had little to do in the village itself. However it was the only police station within a distance of five miles and he had to supervise the whole area. He and his wife and their two sons were well liked and treated with respect by the villagers. There was a feeling of security among the people because of his mere presence, although most of the time it appeared he was only there just in case anything untoward occurred.

The local tailor was a huge man with a large moustache and a strong, deep voice. Most of the children would remember him well for they were all threatened by him if they did not behave. He was the school attendance officer! It was not a pleasant sound to hear his voice at the door asking why an absentee had not been to school!

An important personality in the village was Doctor Rowlands who looked after most of the community and was also the doctor for the quarry at Trefor. He had very pronounced views about when to help and when to pray, and had no use for those who did not help others in a practical way. Doctor Rowlands was born in the county, the son of a slate quarryman. As a young man he wanted to become a doctor and made his way to Glasgow. There he found a job as a postman and succeeded in getting himself registered as a medical student whilst working to keep himself. After he qualified he returned to serve his native county with a charming Scottish nurse as his wife. He had a fine sense of humour and the stories told about him are legion; but above all he will be remembered by the poor of the district, for he often came to their rescue at his own expense. He was not just a doctor but the best type of social worker.

Nant Gwrtheyrn was an isolated little hamlet situated between Yr Eifl and the Irish Sea. In those

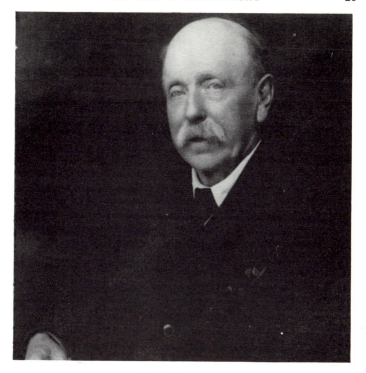

Doctor Rowlands

days it was a thriving village with a granite quarry and five farms in the little valley. There was also a Chapel and a small school. The village was approached from the land by a steep, winding path, its only means of communication with the outside world except by sea. This path was later found to be too difficult even for motor cycle trials. The story is told that the only horse and trap to negotiate this path was driven by a drunken doctor who had been called there for an emergency. He survived the hazardous journey and lived for many years to look after his patients.

William Arthur Jones was the resident Minister

and teacher in this isolated community. He was a stocky little man with dark hair and a squint. He spoke clearly and fluently and many folk have happy memories of the fine work he did as Minister and teacher. In 1916 when home on holiday from the Medical School my father sent me with a friend to see if the farmers were doing all they could to produce food; at the time he was chairman of a committee responsible for this war work in South Caernarfonshire. I found only two farms being worked and a few men at the quarry. The difficulty of getting the granite away by ship and with young people on war service probably accounted for both these changes. Even the two remaining farmers had every intention of leaving as soon as they could.

Long before the First World War, William Arthur Jones left this isolated place and its few remaining people, which no longer justified employing a full time teacher minister, and took over a Church in the busy South Wales mining area of Merthyr Vale. He laboured there for many years but his efforts here again did not prosper. Unemployment and then the 1914-1918 war came and shattered his high hopes.

Finally he came to Bristol to look after the Welsh Presbyterians who held services in John Wesley's famous old Chapel. He was then much older but still filled with enthusiasm for his work. I was pleased to see him after so many years and to speak at his inception meeting. He finished his days in Bristol as also did his wife and son who was a teacher. They were well liked and respected to the last. Throughout his life he was an energetic and enthusiastic leader, kindly and sympathetic but dogged by bad luck. It would have been interesting to have heard from him about his view of life and the whims of fate that help some who do not seem to deserve it but clamp down on others who would appear to merit more success. Envy had no place in his nature. Every member of this little family played its part and left their little world happier for their presence.

Social Life

The centre of our social life at Llanhaelhaearn was the Calvinist Chapel founded by my great grandfather about a hundred and twenty years ago, and he acted as honorary pastor for the last twelve years of his life. It was a sturdy stone building and held about two hundred and fifty people. Two sermons were preached every Sunday, one in the morning and one at the evening service, and Sunday School was held in the afternoon. In winter there was a meeting of the Band

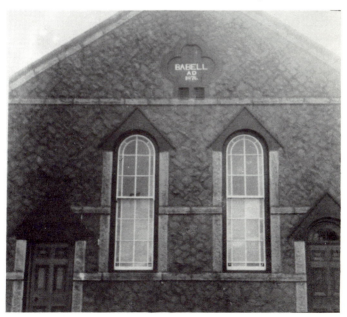

Llanhaelhaearn

of Hope held on one evening of the week for the children. This was presided over by one of the deacons, who was also the singing precentor of the Chapel. I have happy memories of some of these occasions when the more promising of the pupils would demonstrate their skill in tonic sol-fa. In those days there were no musical instruments — only the tuning fork — and it was not till some time later that the Chapel acquired a piano. One evening there was a poorly attended meeting when the singing precentor was absent and one of the old deacons had to have a go at selecting and leading the singing of a tune to suit the words given out by the preacher. Unfortunately this deacon had no ear for music and his two attempts at finding the right tune failed. In despair he called out to a youngster in the audience to "strike the right tune." "Yes, by Gad," said the young man, "I will strike it hard if it comes anywhere near."

There were other meetings during the week and during the year there was a competitive singing meeting — a miniature Eisteddfod — which attracted talent from outside the district. Sometimes small parties of singers or choirs practised for weeks beforehand and often met in secret in a private house if a suitable room could be found. The lack of a village hall or facilities for recreation both indoors and out was very apparent; although, except for the children, there was not much leisure time. The adults worked long hours and their only free time was Saturday afternoon and Sundays.

There was a Chapel House which provided free lodgings for the visiting ministers during the weekend, the expense being borne by the Chapel funds. For about two months of the year free hospitality was given to the visiting preachers by my parents and other farmers in the district. In this way they helped to contribute further to the Chapel funds. My parents always gave a welcome to their particular friends and

I can recall many notable Welsh preachers who stayed
with us. They used to tell us their experiences of the
world outside our little community, read their poetry
and some who had a sense of humour amused us by
recounting their more humorous adventures.

One of our favourite visitors was a preacher who
went under the poetic name of Alafon. He came at
least once a year and on one occasion christened my
young brother Ceiri. On his last visit to us, he was
in a very sad mood. Two catastrophes had happened
to him in one day. Whilst he was digging in his little
garden he heard a shot and immediately his pet robin
had dropped near him, shot in the leg. But what really
brought tears to his eyes was his own carelessness
when he had failed to notice his pet toad in the soil
just in front of him, and he had killed it with his spade.
He wrote a charming poem to its memory.

In those days of the early part of the century there
was a religious revival and Evan Roberts, the
revivalist had a great influence over the whole country.
The Churches and Chapels were full and congregational
singing became extremely popular. Even at our young
age we children thoroughly enjoyed these meeting.

Religious teaching in Sunday School depended very
much on the teacher and some of us used to confuse
one old deacon who was our class teacher and get him
thoroughly mixed up between some of the personalities
of the Old Testament. We brought up specially the
subject of Solomon, Samson and Jonah when these
characters had nothing to do with the lesson of the day,
and he could never remember who was who!

The children of the village were expected to attend
not only Sunday School but also the evening service.
After the sermon was over a meeting of members
followed. The children were then called down to the
front seats and the Minister came down from the
pulpit to ask them to recite the verses they had learnt.
It was our first experience in public speaking — an

opportunity to hear our own voices. We were expected to learn a new verse from the Bible every week. I do not think many parents took an interest in teaching their children (perhaps due to ignorance) but we were more fortunate as our mother took trouble and pleasure in looking up verses for us and I can remember many that I learnt then and can repeat them today.

Welsh was the only language used in the Chapel, and the hymn books and the Bible we used were all written in Welsh.

We did not know very much about the activities of the Church or the Baptist Chapel but there was never any ill feeling between any of the religious sects.

Keeping Sunday as sacred and as a day of rest was of paramount importance in our village and public opinion dictated strict discipline as far as public behaviour was concerned. However, strictness in the home about Sunday observance depended very much on the parents, and on the farm there was always work to be done. Unnecessary work was cut to a minimum and it always seemed a pity, especially at harvest time, that in the summer when weather was so uncertain, all work in the fields stopped on Saturday evening.

The attitude of all farmers in general (and my own father was a good example) to this problem of weather in relation to farm work was conservative. The hay harvest and the corn harvest commenced on a certain date if the weather permitted, but under no circumstances would they start a week earlier even though the weather was good. Their attitude was — 'we have had bad harvests in the past, often because of the weather but on the whole we farmers can trust the Almighty to help us' — a sort of inevitability which has to be borne, although it sometimes helps to have a few grumbles. This attitude extended to animal losses and I can remember my father taking a shot gun and killing a young foal after its mother had broken its leg. There might have been a chance for prevention on all these occasions by a little more foresight, but this might have shown a lack of faith in the Great Power.

I have already mentioned that Welsh was the language of the Chapel, but at school it was different. Our school books at the Board School I attended in the village were all written in English. However, the teachers taught in Welsh and translated the books until the pupil was able to read them for himself. I fear, however, that many a child left school without being able to translate or understand what was written in these books. This was also true of the other two R's although arithmetic and writing were easier to teach. Our school subjects were confined to these three R's for it was as much as the solitary teacher and his pupil teacher (who was his daughter) could cope with. This pupil teacher was screened off in part of the L - shaped room where she could teach the six year olds and under, so that the master could manage the lessons of the older children.

Home Life

To be a parent in a remote country area in those days was a great responsibility. Such a person as a trained midwife or a district nurse did not exist. The friendly neighbour was invaluable, especially if she had had children of her own and had the experience of bringing them up. The notorious, drunken 'mother gamp' found in the big cities was not known in our part of the country and every family had great respect for the two women available who could be called to attend the mothers at the birth of their babies. I have one in mind at the moment of whom my mother thought very highly. I visited her many years later when I was a qualified doctor. She was calm and efficient, very clean and a good cook. There were no hours of duty and she stayed as long as she could be of any help.

She lived in a little cottage on the side of the mountain with a few acres of land where she kept a couple of cows and a pig or two. Her husband worked part time on a near-by farm. They brought up two fine boys, one of whom was killed in a coal mine disaster. The other became a successful carpenter and later a builder in Liverpool. He was very kind to his widowed mother in her old age, but found it very difficult to persuade her to leave her old home and live in the village where she would be near help if needed. When I visited the old cottage, half tumbled down, with my wife during a summer holiday we found that the old lady, well in her eighties, had also decided to visit her tumbled down old home. It was the only occasion when she was unable to insist on our staying for tea and pancakes! But as she said, she could not resist coming back from time to time to see her old home. She must have been over eighty but was as agile as ever.

In case of sickness or accidents there were always many home remedies at hand. There were 'embrocations' for muscular pain, ointments for cuts, warm olive oil for earache and a slice of bacon in flannel tied round the neck for sore throats. Camphorated oil was usually rubbed on the chest for coughs or bronchitis, and a lump of camphor tied up in a small bag round the neck to keep off colds and fleas! For flatulence nothing would do but mushroom ketchup and I remember having to take a spoonful on feeling sick when on a visit to another farm — the relief was instantaneous. The favourite purgative was castor oil and it was even given to us at times as a preventive treatment. I always thought it was worse than the risk of becoming ill. I must not forget to mention goose grease, a most precious commodity, for it was used for so many purposes; for softening the skin when it was chapped and to help keep away the cold when it was well rubbed into the skin. It was also used as dubbin to soften leather of shoes, or straps. 'Oil

Morris Evans' was a universal remedy. It had a powerful 'medicinal' smell and made a fortune for Morris Evans.

Although Dr Rowlands practised in the village, Dr Wynne Griffiths was our family doctor because he had attended our parents and grandparents. However, he lived about eight miles away and had to be fetched by a man on horseback. There was no assurance that he would be at home for he often toured the country in his gig carrying full bottles of various medicines, and might not be home for several days. There was a clear understanding between him and the homes he looked after and parents usually knew what to do until he arrived.

We were all vaccinated against smallpox soon after birth, but my mother insisted on a fresh bottle (tube) being used for each one of us. However, the doctor, knowing us to be of healthy stock, would come a few days later and draw off fluid from the blister for further use as vaccinations. In those days fresh vaccine was not readily available. There were many killer diseases, but of these the worst was diptheria or membranous croup. Then came scarlet fever, tuberculosis, blood poisoning and pneumonia. It must have been a terrifying experience to any parents when they knew what dangers were around the corner and what few remedies they had at hand to meet them.

The duties of the home were many and arduous for houses were not built for labour saving. Washing day was certainly a day of hard labour for a woman with a family. Every drop of water had to be heated over the coal fire, every article scrubbed separately in the tub. Drying the clothes was a terrible problem on wet wintry days in a crowded house. It was a matter of good fortune if the weather came to the rescue.

In most homes a day was set aside for baking bread, another hard task for the mother, but the children usually were able to enjoy the little extra that happened when the oven was heated. Who, at any age can fail to enjoy the delicious smell associated with the baking of bread? All homes did not possess an oven and these depended on the big oven in the village bakery. Three or four days a week were set aside when the large oven would be fired and the villagers allowed to bring their dough, pies and puddings to be cooked. Saturday morning was always a very busy time at the bakehouse. At other times the owner of the oven baked bread for sale. It was very impressive to see the way the big oven was heated — not as it was done at my home with a fire in the grate underneath the oven, but by putting large trays of burning coal in the big iron oven and heating it for a certain time, before withdrawing the fire and putting in the bread or the other food. Some of the bigger farms had these large ovens.

The one acre and a cow type of home meant that meat, milk, eggs and plenty of vegetables were available for the family. Although this meant more work for the mother and sometimes for the older children, what an advantage it had over the town dwellers!

Many of the cottages depended entirely on candles for their lighting, although cheap paraffin lamps were available. For walking around the farm after dark, hurricane lamps were used. When an animal was killed the fat from the carcass was melted down and used for making candles. Two kinds of candles were homemade. Rushes were half peeled and then dipped and soaked in hot fat. When cooled down they could give sufficient light to see one's way around the house and were easy to carry about in special holders. To obtain a thicker and more substantial candle, the wick was cut off a roll and divided into candle lengths. These were then threaded into tin tubes and molten fat poured in, care being taken to keep the wick in the centre of the tube. When solid once more

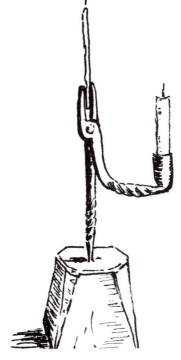

Candle and rush holder

the resulting candle gave a good light. Fires certainly occurred, but everyone knew of this danger and took great care. The causes of fires today from cigarettes, electric wires fusing and pressure oil heaters were unknown then. Coal was plentiful and cheap, but the village was situated far from the coal mines; there was also some wood available. Peat was dug up for our own use on the farm to save coal, but it was not worth the labour of digging and carting away for sale when coal was almost as cheap. I cannot recollect the price of coal in those early days, but even some years later there were occasions when my father bought a truck of about twelve tons for £8 (eight pounds). This had to be carted from the station five miles away.

Warm clothing was of primary importance, to protect the body against the cold inside and outside of the houses. When one realises how little heating there was in the homes and public buildings this need for warm clothing is very obvious. Fashion was forgotten, except on special occasions. Wooden clogs were commonly worn on work days for they were cheap, warm, and kept out the wet. We were all taught that a woollen garment should always be worn next to the skin and any irritation we may have felt was completely ignored. The spinning wheel had fallen into disuse and even the one we had at home was never used, because woollen materials were very cheap. The women did knit for the family, especially long socks and stockings. The only difference between summer and winter dress was that men often discarded their outer woollen vests and coats, for they did not believe in wearing anything but wool next to the skin. On Sundays all the village folk dressed in a dark suit or dress as was befitting that sacred day; they discarded their clogs for leather boots, the men's were usually laced, the women's were buttoned.

The smallness of the cottages helped much to keep them warm as a large fire in the kitchen-living room conveyed warmth to the bed chamber on the ground floor and to the low-ceilinged loft bedroom. No doubt this saved the lives of many old people and of babies during the cold weather. The problem of heating the larger houses was much more difficult and it was no easy matter to keep the spare bedroom properly aired for guests. Copper warming pans filled with hot cinders were placed under the bed and stone hot water bottles, or hot bricks wrapped in flannel were placed between the sheets. Of course the feather bed made a great contribution to maintaining the warmth at night, it also added to the problem of keeping it damp-free when it was not in use.

A considerable number of farm labourers, either unmarried or working some distance away from their homes slept in a loft above the stables. These places would not be tolerated today as fit for human habitation; I remember shuddering at the thought of anyone sleeping on a straw mattress with three or four others in a low-roofed hovel with hardly room to stand a candle. Some of the farms looked after their men better than others, but even on our farm I remember the men preferred to spend their evenings together sitting and smoking their clay pipes on a heap of straw in the stable rather than in the uncomfortable loft. Later, when I was a little older I enjoyed sneaking out to the stable to listen to them discussing the merits of the various animals — horses in particular — and their impressions of the little they knew of the world in general. There was very little comfort for these men, yet strange though it might seem they were happy and enjoyed their life. The simple things like a drink of buttermilk, a cup of tea and chatting together by the light of a hurricane lamp were greatly enjoyed.

Food was cheap in those days — a large loaf for four pence (less than the equivalent of two new pence today) and eggs were sixpence a dozen (the equivalent of two and a half new pence per dozen).

I remember my father selling his first Easter lamb for five shillings — the cost of meat in the butchers' shops was very low compared with the price today. Potatoes cost whatever you liked to pay for them. But if you have no money then everything is expensive. The Poor in the care of the Guardians were given a few shillings a week on which to live. Yet there was a strong community spirit — a concert to help the sick and many a secret visit, to bring gifts. I have tried hard to recollect real misery or a slum dwelling such as I saw many times later on in our big towns, but I cannot.

What a pity that wealth rather than happiness should be the goal of life today!

Looking back at the sort of life the children, myself included, enjoyed seventy years ago, the village, the school and the home was their little world. Discipline was strict but not severe. Lessons were confined to the three R's to which could be added religious teaching in Sunday School. But for most of them the anxiety of examinations did not exist and once school hours ended there was plenty to see and do, especially in the summer time.

The farms at that time were truly family concerns, everyone taking a hand on all occasions to help with the routine work. There was no limit to the age when a child could participate, for even the youngest were found small jobs to do like helping with the sheep or

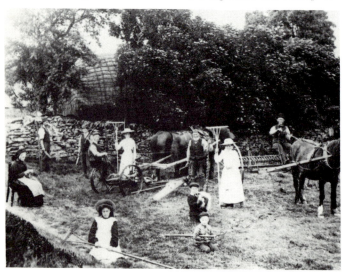

Beginning of hay harvest

taking the milking cows to the field and shutting the gate. As they grew older the tasks became heavier as well as more responsible and they learnt to milk the cows, feed the calves, count the sheep and inspect them for any possible casualties. What a wonderful training that was! Of course they always had the help of a well trained sheep dog to accompany them. These dogs were also useful to keep the foxes away from the poultry which had to be shut in at night.

When I was about six years of age one of my jobs in the early autumn was to walk across the road and up on to the hillside to a stone wall stretching across the mountain. In this high wall was a large hole across which a large flat stone had been rolled to keep the sheep on the mountain for the night. It was my job to roll away this stone and out would come the sheep through the gap and follow me down to the fields where they could have a free run as all the crops had already been harvested.

The village children had none of these responsibilities and were always delighted to be given a chance to help on a farm. One such occasion was in the spring when stones had to be picked up and carried away from the new hayfield so that no damage was done to the mowing machine. For this work a dozen of the older schoolboys were hired on a Saturday for sixpence a day and a good midday meal. They had to collect all the loose stones and throw them into the cart under the supervision of one of the older farm hands.

There was plenty of wild life to be watched and enjoyed even if knowledge of natural history was scanty and had to be picked up by observation.

In the mountain brooks and small streams in the valley many an hour could be spent fishing for tiddlers, usually with a net or a bent pin on the end of a line, or even tickling them. Further down the valley where the rivers were deeper and wider there were plenty of salmon and trout but not for the likes of small village boys! Here, also, were many otters living in the river banks, who were said to rob the rivers of many fish. They were kept in check by a pack of otter hounds famous in South Caernarfonshire known as 'the hounds of Jones Ynysfor'.

Foxes and hares could sometimes be seen on the hills but there were not as many rabbits to be seen round Llanaelhaearn as down in the southern part of the Peninsula. The foxes made ravages on the lambs in the spring, and on the poultry, and the farmers then organised shoots to get rid of them as there was no hunting with packs of hounds anywhere in Caernarfonshire. We always enjoyed watching the dogs giving chase to a hare and usually cornering it in a ditch under a stone wall, but often the hare was much too smart for the dogs and knew how to escape from them.

The mole was another menace to the farmer by disturbing the pasture and the molecatcher was called in periodically. They worked independently and were paid by piece work i.e. by tail, and there was often some doubt that the tails were counted more than once, may be on different occasions elsewhere!

The days when a small boy was put in a field with a rattle to scare away the crows was over, but they were still a menace to the farmer and in spite of scarecrows and shooting managed to get many a good meal from the fields. The loss was very considerable and the farmers usual attitude was to sow a little more to compensate for this. Even so this could hardly make up for the loss. Pigeons were not so abundant and although they did do some damage they were welcomed and shot for pigeon pie! There were always willing hands to feather and dress them ready for the oven.

The only game birds to be found were grouse and a few snipe and wild duck. Some of the older boys became quite skilled with a shotgun.

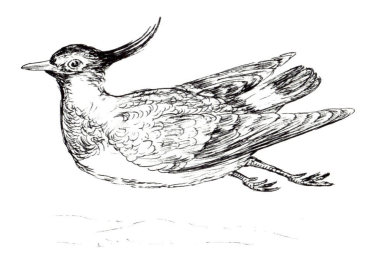

Peewit

Like all country boys we enjoyed looking for birds'
nests, but the lack of hedgerows meant that the nests
had to be found elsewhere. Many of the native birds
were to be found near the hayricks, especially in
winter and spring. These were sparrows, blackbirds,
finches and thrushes and one childish sport was to
place food under a sieve, pull on the string attached
to a stick that supported it and catch the bird. The
bird was then usually released and no harm ever
came to them, but later on this sport was given up
when it was realised that even if it was not cruel it
was certainly unkind.

The peewits' eggs were collected and some boys
even managed to sell them for pocket money. Probably
that is why the cry of the peewit is now seldom heard
in this part of Wales.

The croak of the corncrake was a familiar sound in
the summer. It used to appear in May and disappear

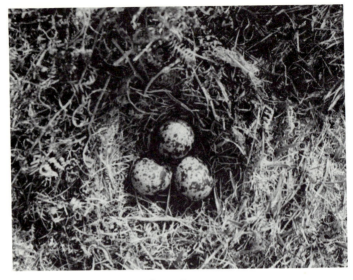

Peewit's nest

in October. Where it went for the winter was a mystery. It was a wily bird and although it did not take to the wing like a pheasant or partridge when disturbed one seldom caught a glimpse of it. Even when the horse-drawn mower was being used in the field and the croak of the bird could be heard, it was difficult to find. If it was caught by the mower it would even feign death but was seldom injured.

There were three favourite small birds popular with most farm boys. They were the robin, the wren and the swallow. We looked with admiration and respect on the robin redbreast. Nothing pleased me more a few years ago than to learn that by public opinion the robin had been chosen as our national bird. The poetic name of my great grandfather was 'Robin Goch' in Welsh. He won the gold medal of the Eisteddfod in Anglesey in 1835 for an Ode on the destruction of Sodom and Gomorrah.' The wren was

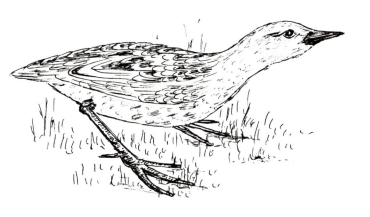

Corncrake

another bird that gave us children much pleasure and excitement to try and find its nest, often in very strange places. When we came to our present house I used to leave an old mackintosh hanging on a peg in the open porch for convenience. One spring I was unable to use the coat because a wren made its nest in the pocket and successfully reared her young. The nest was beautifully built and even had a little hood of dried grass and straw over the top. It was quite a show piece for our visitors. A few days after the baby birds had flown the nest was torn and scattered around in bits. It was out of the reach of a cat or dog and we concluded the wren herself had destroyed it for reasons unknown to us.

The cuckoo was a bird for which we had little respect for we had been taught that from its early days after coming out of the egg it was a cruel bird and a parasite. All the same we enjoyed its song and competed with one another as to who had heard it first and always kept a penny in our pockets in case we heard it. It was difficult to believe that such a beautiful looking bird could have such a cruel nature. One or two late arrivals stayed with us well into the winter but they probably perished from cold.

Finally there were the swallows. They came and went from the middle of April throughout the summer months according to the weather and finally departed at the end of the summer or even earlier if the weather did not suit them. There were always about a dozen swallows' nests that we could see in the cowsheds and when it was time for them to depart, our contingent must have been a strong one. We always believed that information was handed down from one generation to the next and that our visitors, old and young had been with us beforehand and that was why they came again; where they went to in the winter we could only guess, but when the cold snowy weather came along we almost wished that we had been able to go with them.

The blackbirds and thrushes were a nuisance in our somewhat neglected garden where there were a few apple trees, 'bullet plums' and raspberries if we could pick them before the birds. But we did not take this stealing by the birds seriously. There was rhubarb in abundance and we could always pick plenty of bilberries on the mountain in the early summer to be followed by blackberries in the autumn.

As children we little realised how much damage some of the wild animals and birds could do, the pigeons eating our vegetables and the crows enjoying the corn. We had not learnt that there was a conflict between man and wild life for survival. We just enjoyed exploring the countryside with its wild inhabitants.

About the time when school was over in July, the bilberries would be ready for gathering. The children would then go in parties bilberrying on the hillside or along the banks beside the lanes. It was a tiring job and often more were eaten than went into the basket, but they made delicious tarts and jam. Later the blackberries waited to be picked and they too were a welcome addition to the food store.

There was none of the excitement of radio or television for dark winter evenings but I do not remember any complaint of boredom from the children. There were always books to read or stories to be listened to, told by their elders, either true or imaginary.

There were very few musical instruments to be found in the district so that any pleasure in music for the children was in singing. They also learnt to recite and tell stories. They shared very freely the entertainment supplied by the older folk both at home and at the Chapel. All public entertainments had to be held at the Chapel as there was no other suitable building. The programme therefore had to be chosen carefully for the sacred place. There is little doubt that the experience gained by the children in singing, reciting and speaking before an audience was very valuable to many of them later in life.

Life in our 'New' Villages, 1905 ...

When we moved to my second home, another farm situated between the two villages of Llannor and Efailnewydd, the landscape was entirely different and the villages themselves had a very different character from Llanaelhaearn. The fields were bounded by hedges instead of stone walls and spread out over the flat countryside. There were more trees along the roadside, and more copses and woods in the district than on the hilly slopes of Yr Eifl. There were more cattle and dairy herds to be seen, fewer sheep and many of the fields were used for growing corn and root crops.

Efailnewydd is on the main road from Nefyn to Pwllheli where it is joined by a road coming from the south west of the Peninsula. Although there were more short terraces of old stone cottages there were also houses that had been built more recently and the village had developed at a much later date than Llannor. There were two shops and an old mill, but because it was less than two miles from a busy market town and on a good main road the villagers were able to do a great part of their shopping in the town. There was a village pub at the junction of the two main roads.

Llannor, on the other hand was the 'capital' of the parish. It was an old village with a Parish Church, a cemetery and school at its centre. The children from the surrounding farms and hamlets and from Efailnewydd all attended Llannor school until they were old enough to go to the secondary school in Pwllheli. It was a Church School at Llannor and it was fortunate to have good headmasters, young men of whom at least two became prominent figures in the Church after leaving the School.

Besides the Church there was a small Chapel and a post office as well as a village Inn. But it was a quiet little village only disturbed by the noise of the children in the playground or arriving and leaving school each day. There were services held in the Church and Chapel on Sundays and at other times for weddings and funerals.

Probably because of its more accessible position Efailnewydd was the centre for social life and this was chiefly connected with the Chapel and its activities. There was not the same community spirit that existed at Llanaelhaearn for the villagers could look to Pwllheli for their social interest and market days when they could buy and sell. All the same there were characters amongst them who were well known either for the part they played in public life or for their eccentricities.

At the junction of our byroad with the main road from Pwllheli to Nefyn were three small cottages called Ty'nlon. The end house towards Nefyn was on the main road, though entered by a door from the side. The other two had a low stone wall with a paved path about five feet in width between the house and the wall. This stone wall was of immense importance to the inhabitants of these two cottages for on fine summer evenings they and their friends could carry on their chats whilst sitting or leaning on the wall and at the

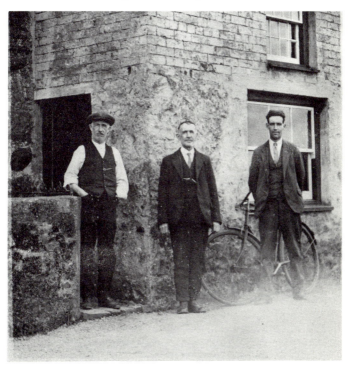

One of the tailors with his assistants

same time watch the people and traffic passing along the main road. Hardly ever did a passer-by fail to stop and have a word or two and even the driver of a horse and trap would pull up for a chat.

That wall could almost be called the headquarters of the 'bush telephone' system of the district for it was amazing how news reached there from all corners of the countryside. When I first knew it, the end house consisted of two low rooms — one up and one down with a small space for cooking at the back. The privy and the water supply were both in the garden to the rear at the far end of a paved path. The husband was a gardener and a keen fisherman in his spare time. His fat old wife kept a sweet shop which could never have brought her much profit for she always gave us a 'little extra' for our pennies. They had a daughter and all three slept upstairs and lived in the little all-purpose room downstairs. After a time, however, they moved away and the cottage was taken by tailors who lived next door but one.

They were two partners named Jones and Davies. Owen Jones, a short, heavy man with a leg in irons was the 'chairman of the board' in spite of the fact that Davies, the smaller and nimbler partner kept the accounts and looked after the pony and trap in which they went about the countryside when required. There was never a dull moment in the workshop. If there was not a customer or a gossip or both with them, the tailors always had something to recount or an amusing anecdote to recite. Sometimes there was a lull in the conversation and a simple swear word would come from the assistant who was working in the loft. Out would come Owen Jones' big stick and he would bang it on the ceiling which he could reach from where he and Davies sat cross legged on the big table in the window. Owen Jones was deacon and could not possibly approve of such language; but we thought that these little episodes were more amusing than the local gossip and I am sure Owen Jones enjoyed them! I have very happy memories of these tailors who made the clothes for all our family — they made my suits for nearly twenty years. Owen Jones also cut my hair for many years without payment. He was quite up to date with his clippers and for some of his special clients he finished off with a singe.

The mole catcher lived in a small cottage with one or two paddocks, hardly big enough to be called a smallholding. His name was Francis Longer and was thought to have emigrated from Yorkshire. He spoke neither Welsh nor English properly, but could be understood. We always regarded him as a real expert at his job and admired him, because he could even catch the moles alive. It is said that if he had a grudge against any near-by farmers he would take the live moles and dump them in their fields. I wonder if that was true?

There was a very good story told of Francis Longer which must have been true for I heard it many times. It was a hot summer's day and as usual he had taken his little produce from the garden and the poultry, and possibly some dairy produce from his cow, to the market, where he is purported to have had too much to drink. He had to walk home a distance of over four miles and though it was difficult to guess his age, he was certainly no youngster. On his way back he had to pass through the village and was seen by Mary Jones to be walking unsteadily and carrying a basket on his arm. She also noticed that he was hatless, considered a disreputable state for any man in those days. To her it could only mean he was drunk. The bush telephone came into action and the message reached the ears of the Chapel authorities where Francis Longer attended and at whose services he often took part. A court of enquiry was set up and Francis was summoned before the deacons (at that time there was no minister). He duly turned up and the witness, Mary Jones was called. Francis was allowed to cross-question her and although I only have it on hearsay his cross-questioning would have done credit to many a successful lawyer to whom I have since listened in court. The outcome of the enquiry was that Francis Longer was proved innocent and that he was merely hot and tired and was carrying his hat in his basket. Under the circumstances he was let off. This episode shows how strict some of these small Chapels were in the matter of alcoholic drink and drunkenness.

There were many other amusing characters living in this district. Several of the well known and respected families in the neighbourhood had inter-married, but in spite of this I was never aware of any trouble or jealousies arising between the parents or the children. Family discipline was excellent, and I cannot recollect the need for a village constable and there was not one in the whole parish!

In the village lived two well known singers; John Hughes the baritone, and the tenor William J. Hughes. John Hughes was very musical and was precentor at the local Chapel. William the tenor had a marvellous voice but his knowledge of music was limited. He later married Leila Megan, a famous operatic singer. Under the leadership of John Hughes the two men hardly ever failed to win duet competitions in Eisteddfods all over North Wales. On one occasion an adjudicator who did not know their background, referred in his comments to the remarkable influence of the good tenor on the baritone! A serious blow to poor John and he took the criticism very much to heart.

The old miller and his wife were prominent members of the Chapel. He was a short, heavily built man in his late middle age. Mrs Williams, his wife, was English but had learnt Welsh which she spoke with many a gap and in a strange accent. She had become influenced by the recent religious revival and took part in the prayer meetings. It was said that on one occasion during a Sunday morning service she was praying aloud and in the middle of her prayer she stopped and exclaimed, "The Devil has just told me that my dinner is burning in the oven. I tell him before you all — eat it then." My best recollection of the old man was at the end of a Sunday school lesson. The class was being questioned on the lesson of the Prodigal Son. One of the questions asked by the deacon in charge was what were the husks to which the verse referred? Charles Pritchard, a real old Christian who was very knowledgeable on the Bible and its commentaries answered that it was the food given to the swine in those Eastern lands. The deacon asked for any other suggestions and the miller replied, "Yes, they were the sweepings from the floor of the mill." The natural response of a miller!

A man who had lost a leg whilst working on a farm was eking out an existence on a meagre compensation. His name was John Jones, a short sturdily built man whose tall, thin wife wore glasses and always looked half-starved. I have never met anyone who could exaggerate as much as he did. He could turn a small incident into almost a miracle. He used to wander into our fields at harvest time and we all had great fun listening to his stories. I knew they could not be true but this no doubt, helped me in my journey through life to discriminate between the probable and the impossible. The workers in the field were never very pleased to see him for he was very free with his advice which usually did not agree with their routine. One of his boastful stories about his great strength (for my father had told me how strong he had been before his accident) was how, when in Liverpool he had picked up a sack of hobnails and lifted it on to a cart after several men had struggled and given up the effort. He even said that the imprints of his boots on the pavement are to be seen to this day. He derived much pleasure in the telling, and one little episode could be the subject of a long discourse. This also applied to his impromptu prayers. The boys of the village enjoyed listening to him at his evening prayers at the door of his little cottage, but when they thought he had been at it long enough they tapped at the door and ran away.

No account of Efailnewydd during the first quarter of this century would be complete without a short account of Bob John. He was the eldest son of a family of five. His father was a quarryman who, from being an uncertain character, as the result of the religious revival in the early part of the century became a pillar of the little Chapel and remained so until the end of his days. There was no industry in any of the little villages around and those who did not want to work on the farms were employed largely in the Gimlet quarry at Pwllheli. Transport was difficult and they had to find their way to work by walking or cycling to the quarry or outlying farms, often a distance of three or four miles. Walking, of course, was no hardship but time to them was precious and for that reason, throughout the land the bicycle became a necessity. In a temporary shed in the village Bob John set up his cycle store and repair shop and his fame spread far and wide. Not only was he a skilled worker but he showed much kindness and consideration for all his clients amongst whom were numerous children who had to find their own way to school in those days. His younger brother, Owen, became a racing cyclist and was hardly ever beaten. The cycle track in the Recreation ground at Pwllheli gave him and several others opportunity to practice and compete in races. He was killed in the First World War.

When we returned to practise in the district in 1924 Bob John had established a large motor garage at Pwllheli and there he dealt extensively with motor cycles and cars. I had had some prewarning of this new venture when with two friends he came up to London to attend the Motor Show. He was taken ill, suffering from a nasty boil and he found himself a casualty at the Outpatient department of the Middlesex Hospital. It so happened in that particular year, 1920, I was the Casualty Officer. It gave me not only the opportunity to treat him but to give him lunch and to have a long chat with him. It was from him that we acquired our two bull-nosed Morris Cowleys for the practice four years later. He had two daughters and seven sons four of whom are still carrying on with the business.

An old friend Mr Richard Elias Pritchard once told me that if you want to make a success of a business which is concerned with service to people it is essential to find a place where there are plenty of people. He had moved to London and established a large and very successful catering business in the capital. Bob John had all the qualities which would have made for great success and if there had been enough people around, who knows but that we might have had another Lord Nuffield from Efailnewydd!

Looking back in my book of memories is not unlike the experience felt by the poet Thomas Gray when he was sitting in a country Churchyard but, unlike the poet I knew some of the folk during their lifetime. Some whom I can remember from my early days at Llanaelhaearn are buried in the village Churchyard. Of those I recall when we had moved to my second home some are in the Churchyard at Llannor and others are buried in the Chapel cemetery at Penrhos where my own parents rest. They did not acquire fame nor were they filled with worldly ambitions, neither did they show any sign of jealousy or ill will. They lived and played their part in life working hard and trying their best to be a burden to no one.

"Far from the madding crowd's ignoble strife,
Their sober wishes never learned to stray;
Along the cool sequester'd vale of life
They kept the noiseless tenor of their way."

Surely their souls deserve a better memorial than they had in this world. They must survive whatever the scientific mind may think.

Scattered round the village were several small farms and one or two large ones. Farming in those days consisted of looking after sheep, a few milking cows and butter making, ploughing up the land where possible with horse ploughs, planting potatoes and sowing seeds of corn, swedes and mangolds for animal feed during the winter. Two of the busiest times on the farm that I remember well were harvest and sheep shearing. It was a laborious life for the farmer and his wife — at least twelve hours a day for the farmer and fifteen for the wife — seven days a week. Money was very scarce; a good farm hand's wage was from £6 to £10 a half year with board and lodging. When my parents were my age, they told me, that the best man in the neighbourhood — and he was second to none — earned eight golden sovereigns every half year. One very good worker on our farm insisted on having a week's holiday every six months. He dressed himself in his Sunday best and went to a Beddgelert hotel for the week until his money was exhausted and after that he was ready for another six months hard labour. Needless to say he was a bachelor.

The machine age had not arrived and the only farm machinery in those days were the two-wheeled carts with extension for carrying hay, sledges for stone work on the mountain slopes, the hay mower and a wide horse-drawn hay rake. Petrol had not yet arrived. The farmer had to depend on horses for power and there were several teams of fine horses to

be seen and a few ponies for pulling the machinery.
Overturning the cart and smashing the shafts was not
an uncommon experience on the hill farms and this
happened more than once without much harm to horse
or man, but considerable damage to both cart and
harness.

There was a story told about Owen Jones, a well
known cloth mill owner who used to attend market at
Pwllheli every Wednesday. He had a distance of
twenty miles to travel and had to leave home with his
pony and light cart in the early hours of the morning.
He acquired the first 'old Ford' to arrive in the
district and this saved him a considerable amount of
time. But it also took him some time to acquire the
necessary skill to drive, although there were no
driving tests in those days, and it took him longer
still to forget some of his old habits. He always
saluted every one on the way and in doing so took his
eyes off the road — at very little risk in those days
of no traffic and slow speeds — then he would quickly
return to his steering. On one occasion, however,
while going along a country lane, he saw going in the
same direction a wide horse-drawn hay rake taking
up all the lane with a man leading the horse and
another with a small wooden rake on his shoulder
walking behind. Owen Jones driving along behind
realised he could not pass. He shouted and the driver
drew the rake well up the hedge but there was still no
room to pass. Owen Jones put his head out and
shouted, " I shall run into you — I can't help it. " The
man behind the rake ran back and shouted, "Why the
hell don't you stop?" "Well, yes, " said Owen Jones,
"I never thought of that!" He did manage to stop and
there was no accident. When they were learning to
drive all my children heard this story several times.
There would be far fewer accidents on our roads
today if drivers remembered that they can always
stop and wait.

Farm Life

Plenty of hand tools were always available and well kept ready for use — the scythe, the spade, the pitchfork and the sickle with its little two-pronged wooden fork companion and the fork with a bent end for pulling the manure from the cart. A more interesting occupation for us children was to use a little hand turner with which they twisted straw and hay into ropes for keeping the matting down over the hay and corn ricks until there was time to thatch; these ropes then formed part of the thatching.

The cows were brought into the cowshed twice a day to be milked by hand. Although the milker was supposed to wash his hands and the cow's udders, there was no running water in the building so the udders were just dry cleaned before the milk was drawn off into a bucket and then emptied into the churn. If the milk was to be made into butter or cheese it was carefully filtered when it reached the dairy and poured into large earthenware jars. The rest of the milk was sent by cart to the villages and ladled out by the pint into jugs at the various houses.

There was always a certain amount of mechanical power available on the farm, although the horse was by far the most valuable to assist human effort with the farm work. The water-wheel at my first home was situated by the side of the dairy, which was a stone built single-room wing of the house. The control of the water-wheel always fascinated me. There were two fairly large pools, one situated above the other on sloping fields above the house. A small brook ran into the top pool and the overflow as well as the water from the outlet ran into the lower pool. The outlet of the top pool had to be blocked by dropping a steel plate into position and leaving it in that position until the bottom pool was empty. Then this steel plate had to be lifted up by hand to allow the water to flow into the lower pool. Control of the flow from the lower

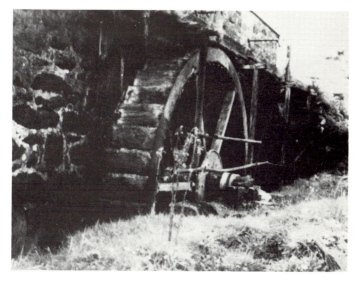

Water-wheel

pool was by a lever connected by a wire to a similar plate at the outlet of the pool. So the plate could be raised or lowered as required from the building. It was very important that this mechanism should be carefully maintained. From the outlet the water was carried along an open wooden channel to the top of the water-wheel, which was also made of wood. When the wheel rotated it emptied itself into a wide drain built under the yard and into a ditch in the field below. On the other side of the dairy were the machines operated by the water power; one for chaff cutting, another for cutting up gorse and one for chopping up roots such as swedes and mangolds. These latter were mixed with hay or straw for feeding the animals. There was a lever to control the outflow of water from the lower pool, both in the dairy and in the farm building. The water-wheel was connected by pulleys and belts to the machinery: the churn in the dairy was operated by the same means. It was essential that in the case of accidents, particularly with machines in the farm buildings there should be a quick break in the connection with the water power. First the belt of the machine was thrown on to a free wheel pulley and then the water-wheel itself was stopped by opening a trap door in the wooden channel to the water-wheel to allow the water to flow into a ditch at the top of the yard. This trap door was usually kept open when the wheel was not in use. In summer time and against mother's instructions, I spent many happy hours playing 'boats' in this little brook. My feet were always wet and all my colds were blamed on this! I do not think my father was of an engineering turn of mind otherwise he would have done as two bachelor uncles had done on their farm. They had built a battery house, charged the batteries from the water-wheel and wired the house and farm buildings for lighting.

We had the great advantage over some farms in having gravity to drive the water to give us power, but when we moved to our second home we had to adopt a method used by other farms of having a pony to pull a pole to turn a wheel by walking round and round, and this wheel was connected to machines in the farm buildings. Many hours I spent sitting on the long pole pulled by the pony to make sure it did not stop while churning or other machine-driven work was in progress. It was a great relief when the oil engine replaced all this in about 1909. In some of the smaller farms large dogs turned the wheel on a sloping platform but we looked upon this as cruel and there was considerable public outcry against it.

It has always seemed a pity that more use was not made of wind as a power to help on farms and in the home. Windmills are seen very frequently on the continent of Europe and in this part of Wales we have never been lacking in strong winds. In only a few farms was a windmill to be seen and even then it was only used to drive water from a well to supply tanks for farm and domestic uses. In those days farmers had very little engineering skill and maybe the attention needed to maintain the windmill was somewhat of a deterrent. Also in the hilly districts there was plenty of water and gravity to produce power. There were many hand pumps to obtain water from a well or spring, and to operate these was not considered a heavy task for either man or woman. It was surprising that more use was not made of piping to carry water to supply tanks whence gravity would do the rest. No doubt the obstacle to this was the cost of installing such a system and the farmers and their helpers were lacking in knowledge of plumbing and were usually tenant farmers.

Before the arrival of oil or petrol, farming therefore depended on four sources of power — five if one includes man. They were the dog, the horse, water and wind.

Most villages had their mill where the corn was ground. In our village the mill was situated a few hundred yards down the hill and had a very efficient water power working the water-wheel. The grinding was done with grooved millstones rotating on each other and this process could be adjusted to grind the corn finely or coarsely as required. The old miller was a well-known personality. He had five donkeys to carry bags of corn, the team led by one of his sons. It was a great treat for the boys to see Twm, his son, walking by the side of the team of five donkeys, cracking his whip. On the way back they trotted along with Twm sitting on the leader. It was difficult to recognise the old miller in his Sunday suit as the same man when he had been covered in flour all the week.

Oats and barley were the two crops grown in our part of the country. Very little was sold, because nearly all was used for feeding purposes. Some of the grain was taken to the mill to be ground and the flour was used for making barley bread, which was the main type of loaf used. White bread was not often eaten, because wheat flour was expensive or the loaves themselves would have to be bought. Oats, on the other hand were treated differently from barley; some was used for animal feeding, but the oats required for human needs were sent to the mill where they were first baked in a special brick-lined kiln until the kernels (glume) were separated out. They were then sifted from the husks and were ready for use. With this, oatmeal cakes were made and I can remember many dishes with Welsh names, such as 'brwas', 'llymru' and 'sucan', but alas, I have been unable to find English translations for these words. They were very tasty and nutritious, but have fallen into disuse for many years and I could not possibly try to describe the way in which they were made.

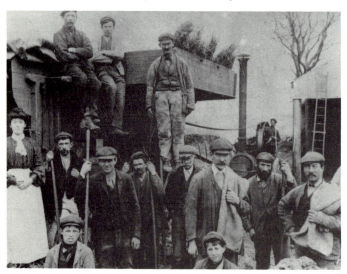

Threshing machine

The day the threshing machine arrived at the farm was a very important one. Perhaps it was not such a social occasion as corn harvest or shearing, but it was a time of great fun for the children and of feasting for the workers. Preparations for the day had started some weeks before, because the threshing machine had to be booked and the neighbours who were coming to help or send their men, had to be told. The machine consisted of two parts — the actual thresher and the steam engine. The power was transferred from the engine through a fly wheel and belt to the wheel of the thresher. Both machines rested on their own four iron wheels. Usually only one day was given to threshing and that was soon after the harvest; some of the corn was left to be threshed later in the autumn. The requirements varied with the size of the farm. The engine was coal fired so it was important to see that there was plenty of coal. It was just as well that coal was cheap for a ton lasted no time in the greedy oven of the steam engine. When all was ready on the farm, the machine had to be fetched from where it had last been in use, and this required two teams of horses. Two men came with the machine to set it up and operate it. This was done by first adjusting the distance from each other and then stabilising them, ready to be used when the threshing day arrived. It was then necessary to light a fire to generate the steam so that the engine could start working in the early hours of the following day.

Then the great day started and I have a vivid picture in my mind of a little man on top of the thresher spreading a sheaf of corn into the machine after it had been passed from the rick through various hands to his assistant to cut the binding and hand it to him. The other operator who had travelled with the machine kept an eye on the engine and the steam; he would relieve his partner from time to time on top of the thresher. It was the duty of one man, usually super-

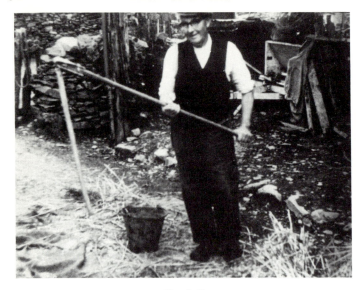

The flail

vised by my father, to watch the grain coming through
the graded chutes to the sacks. These were then
carried to the corn loft and emptied into bins. All this
meant a great deal of dust and it was surprising to see
how few of the men were affected by this dust, whereas
I sneezed without stopping and had to keep as clear from
the grain chutes as I possibly could. When the rick was
nearly empty there was plenty of excitement to be had
watching the dogs hounding out and destroying the rats
which had come to spend the winter in the rick. By
far the biggest harvest of rats was gathered when the
second threshing occurred at the end of the winter.
In those days rats could only be destroyed with the
help of dogs — trapping or shooting could not possibly
cope with the problem.

Some smallholders still used the old-fashioned
method of threshing the grain by using flails to
separate the grain from the straw. Usually husband

and wife worked together. They spread the sheaf of corn in thin layers over a large canvas and brought the flails down sharply on the corn. It was a laborious job, especially for the woman, but the smallholder did not have sufficient corn to justify hiring the threshing machine.

Much good Welsh poetry has been composed as tributes to the dog and his qualities as man's best friend. Eifion Wyn, the famous local poet with his long experience as a shepherd composed some beautiful verses to his dog Mot. I only wish I could translate them into English without sacrilege. One thing is certain, that man would indeed be helpless to look after a flock of sheep without the help of at least one dog. I do not remember in my youth seeing any sheep dog trials such as are common today, but I do remember seeing and hearing of some outstanding feats performed by dogs showing higher intelligence than some human beings. In my old home near Yr Eifl there were several dogs and I used to watch my father with his shepherd's crook going with Lassie and never failing to pick out a lamb or a sheep to examine it. I always marvelled at the way the dogs understood commands given to them by whistling. The son of the farmer who followed us when we left my first home told me a remarkable story. He had come to visit his father. Looking across the valley at his own farm he saw a flock of sheep crossing from the moorland into his cornfield. He put his fingers to his mouth and whistled. His dog appeared on the wall in front of his house; he whistled again and the dog turned round, went straight to the cornfield and drove the sheep back to the moorland. He whistled yet again to tell the dog that all was well and I suppose the dog took this as a word of thanks. The distance to his farm was about half a mile as the crow flies or as the sound of a whistle travels!

On another occasion I remember getting up in the

early hours of the morning to walk three or four miles
with two uncles to collect the sheep for shearing. We
climbed up the mountain accompanied by three dogs
and we collected the sheep from these hundreds of
acres of mountain within a few hours. Of course the
dogs did the work while my uncles whistled their
commands. All the sheep were then brought down to
the fold and examined to see if they were fit to travel.
Those that were not fit were put into the inner fold to
separate them and left there until they could be dealt
with. It had been a wonderful day for picnicking and
we arrived back in the evening with several hundred
sheep.

The dogs again are invaluable when the sheep are
brought off the mountain in the autumn to be sorted —
some to be sold, some to be taken back to the mountain
in the spring and some to be fattened on the farm for
sale later. When this sorting was being carried out it
was most important that some of the older sheep (not
necessarily the oldest) should be returned to that part of
of the mountainside from whence they came, for they
knew their own territory and hardly ever trespassed on
their neighbours. These older sheep formed a nucleus
in each area and taught the younger ones to know their
territory. I have never noticed sheep fighting over
their rights to a particular area as robins do so
noisily around the house.

It was not with sheep alone that the dog was so
useful. One old bitch of ours used to know the time to
fetch the cows in for milking and would seek the
assistance of anyone who happened to be near by to
open the gate for her. As watch dogs they were the
most useful to guard against foxes and other vermin.
If there are two or three of them together they make a
formidable army against unwanted intruders. There
was one very sad occurrence when an otherwise good
sheep dog was led astray by a 'rogue' dog to hunt
down sheep and lambs. Often this 'rogue' dog was an

outsider, but sometimes even a trained farm dog could become a 'rogue'. The only way to deal with such a dog was to kill it, for once it had acquired a taste for killing sheep it could never be trusted again. In a sheep farming area all dogs had to be kept under control, for they could do much damage to a flock, especially on a moonlight night during the lambing season.

Dogs were not the only culprits that killed or maimed young lambs. Crows also viciously attacked them, especially if they had strayed away from their mothers. Farmers were constantly waging war against this enemy.

Social events important to farmers and their families and to the country folk in general were the Fairs, which were held in the villages and towns. The 'hiring fairs' were held twice a year in the main towns and

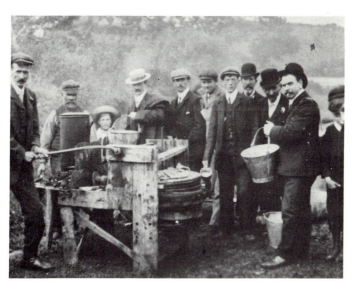

Preparing for a picnic — tea-making

here the workers, both men and women were engaged
(and sometimes re-engaged) for six months till the
next hiring fair.   The terms of the contract were
decided and the date on which work would start.
Usually the men and women expected a few days'
holiday before beginning the new contract as it would
probably be the only holiday they would get in six
months.   The contract was a verbal one and sealed
with a sixpenny piece. The afternoon of fair day was
given over to spending some of the hard-earned money
on drink, fun fairs and sweethearts.   Several Cheap-
jacks came to the fair and set up their wares. They
sold everything, from cheap clothing, goldfish,
coconuts and patent pills to medicines that would cure
any ills.   There were coconut shies, shooting ranges,
and roundabouts with plenty of raucous music. For the
children it was always a special occasion and we
enjoyed every moment till it was time to go, and then
we envied the town youngsters who had not got the long
tramp home.

   The other fairs held in the villages ended the day
like the hiring fairs, but they started very differently.
The cattle and the horses were led along the road to
where the sales were to be held. Here the dealers,
mostly from England came to make their offers.
Sometimes interpreters were called in to help with
the deals, but the sellers usually had a clear knowledge of the values.   Some dealers had a trick of
wandering along the road to meet the farmer and his
animals, before he had a chance of discussing prices
with others, but the bush telegraph was quite efficient
and the dealers' tricks seldom brought them a bargain.

   On market day in Pwllheli there were usually farm
carts in the square and much squealing from the
many little pigs that had been brought for sale.   In
the market hall were stands set aside for the farmers'
wives to sell their produce — butter, eggs, chickens
and garden produce.   There were always plenty of

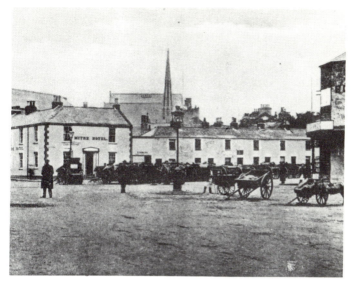

Market day in Pwllheli – little pigs in cart

eager buyers and an air of bustling activity.

Animal Health

One of the great problems that every farmer has
had to face over the years is the question of animal
health. With the great advance in recent years in
bacteriology, biology and epidemiology it has been
possible to give much greater economic security to
the farmer in this respect, but at the end of the last
century they had to depend much more on their own
and their neighbours' knowledge of the methods to
deal with sickness and accidents to their livestock.
Some farmers who were descended from old farming
families had accumulated much useful information on
how to deal with these problems and, indeed, how
they might prevent the occurence of some of them.
But on the whole, there was a great lack of general

knowledge of this important aspect of stock farming.

When I was a visiting Professor to Yale University in 1956 the Historical Library was disposing of their 'unwanted books' and, partly from curiosity I had a look at the stall. I picked up a small leather-bound book and took it to the attendant. She said at once, "You can take that — we just do not know what it is all about." I thanked her very much and took it away. I have it before me as I write. It is a book published in 1816 by John Edwards from Dyffryn Clwyd and re-printed in Utica in 1849. Utica, in the State of New York was at that time the stronghold of the Welsh community in the United States. The title of the book, written in Welsh is 'Advice from experience to all animal owners about cows, calves, oxen, horses and sheep, how to recognise disease and the most effective way of treating them'.

I have read much of this little book and in many respects it is remarkably up to date, although written over a hundred and fifty years ago. I have tried to summarise and translate some of the points made by John Edwards:

1.   My grandfather and my father had long experience of dealing with healthy and sick animals and I accompanied them whenever I could, watched them carefully and listened to their reasoning.

2.   I have studied many books on this subject of animal sickness and have come to the conclusion that much has been written by men with no practical experience. The English have had more experience than the Welsh in these matters.

3.   You will have noticed that I have often

omitted to mention local herbs and leaves from my recipes. I have done this on purpose not because they have no value, but because of the general ignorance on such matters. It is safer to purchase the materials required from a reliable shop or stall.

4. I have seen many trying to save money or trouble and not doing the job properly or not giving the correct dose at the right time. That may mean a long illness for the animal and so more expense, or even failure of the treatment altogether.

5. Cleanliness is always most important for external wounds. Wash and clean the wound not only to remove the poison, but to keep the healthy part free from disease. Watch the dog dealing with his wounds, you cannot compete with him and his wound heals quickly. Cover the wound with a clean dressing of soft material not too tightly or too slack. If these instructions are followed the type of medicinal application is not important.

What a wonderful clinical teacher John Edwards would have made in a Medical school!

About the end of the last century there was a local boy who, after private study, succeeded in gaining an entry to the Edinburgh Veterinary School. There he qualified as a Veterinary Surgeon and later obtained the F.R.C.V.S. London. After qualifying he returned to his native heath at the beginning of this century. His name was Roberts — 'Roberts the Vet' as he was

usually called and he set up his surgery in Pwllheli.
He was an outstanding person in every respect and
made some notable contributions to the advancement
of veterinary science. He was followed in the practice
by his son who, however, died in the prime of his life,
but the practice is still continuing in other hands. Of
course it was more than 'Roberts the Vet' could
manage to cover 200 square miles of farming country
and so the farmers had to depend a good deal on their
own and their neighbours' knowledge and assistance.

When I look at the picture I have in my mind of these
small rural communities at the beginning of the century
I note their difficulties and their problems. Nevertheless, what stands out most vividly is the unruffled
manner in which they faced their inevitable day to day
responsibilities. Such an attitude today does not satisfy
those who want change for its own sake calling it
progress. There was quiet satisfaction when success
crowned their efforts. In a closely knit community
their joys and sorrows could be shared; also examples
were there for them to follow. Their roots were there
and their forbears had 'fought the good fight'. There
is little doubt that the way in which they faced up to
life's problems brought out their best qualities.

II. BETWEEN THE GREAT WARS

"Mae byd a bywyd oll yn bethau gwerth chweil,
Ac mae cadw bywyd yn fyw yn ddyletswydd a ddeil."

"Life is for living and worthwhile, that's true,
And the keeping of life alive is our due."

Sir Thomas Parry Williams.

Pwllheli in 1925

Joan and I left Bristol in January 1925, and came to
Pwllheli to start general practice. We found a
conveniently situated house in the centre of the town,
and we acquired two small 12 H.P. Morris Cowley
cars to take us about the country.

Neither of us knew much, and nothing from
experience, of life in a small Welsh country market
town. It is true that for five years I had cycled daily
through the town to the county school, and many of my
fellow pupils were from the town itself; but I seldom
visited it except for shopping, and knew little of the
life of the town children out of school. It was therefore an entirely new experience for us both to live in
Pwllheli.

Pwllheli was a borough and had a population of less
than three thousand, but it was really much more than
that — it was the 'capital' of a rural area of about

two hundred square miles. For all special occasions in the district such as the National Eisteddfod, Y Sassiwn (denominational preaching meetings), singing meetings and concerts, as well as agricultural fairs, the town was chosen as the centre. It also had the advantage of being the railway terminus. Wednesday of every week was market day. On all these occasions the people of South Caernarfonshire flocked here, and they looked upon the town as their capital.

The old town itself was half a mile from the sea, and the land near the beach had been developed for residential purposes. What little industrial development there was, apart from that connected with the sea, had taken place in the town centre.

If it had not been for a very efficient railway service in the early part of the century Pwllheli and the whole of the Llŷn Peninsula would have been 'land-locked'. No wonder there had been agitation to have the line extended as far as Nefyn to help still further the transport problem of the rural area, but this never materialised.

The London and North Western Railway from Euston through Chester and Bangor came as far as Afonwen junction about five miles away and there it joined the Cambrian Railway, thus connecting the Cardigan Bay coast with the northern part of the county. The Cambrian Railway was later absorbed by the Great Western, and, as might be expected, the local service did not improve as far as the requirements of the local people were concerned. Of course there was as before, a direct link between Pwllheli, the Midlands and London. Llŷn depended almost entirely on rail transport for its supplies of artificial fertilisers, lime and coal for the farmers, as well as other materials for the traders. Transport of animals was made easier. Cattle, sheep and pigs from the agricultural areas were able to reach the English markets quickly. This meant better prices for the farmers and made them less dependent on the dealers. The economic value of the railway therefore was very much appreciated. Times had certainly changed from the last century when the animals had to be 'walked' long distances to get to market, often resulting in considerable losses. Even now some were walked to the station or local markets, but many were transported in horse drawn carts adapted for this purpose.

The Gimlet rock — once an island — was a landmark, especially to the sailors out in the bay. It covered five acres and was a hundred feet high. When ship-building in Pwllheli declined, the Gimlet granite quarry which had started in 1837 with the building of a landing stage, became more important and soon employed several hundred men. It produced setts for paving the streets of the big towns of England and Wales and at one time these were in great demand. When, however, these towns started using tarmacadam instead of setts the quarry changed over to producing chippings. These chippings for tarmacadam were the quarry's main product in 1925. The old rock was gradually being used up and many folk dreaded the thought that this old landmark would disappear altogether.

There were several hotels and public houses in the town, and they provided stables for the horses and traps on market days and at other times. In view of the attitude of the Chapels to the drink question there were also temperance hotels and eating houses. An amusing story is told of a prominent citizen who went for a short holiday to Llandrindod Wells — the Spa was very popular with the people of the district — but failed to find a room at his usual temperance place and had to be satisfied with one at a licensed hotel. At dinner on the first evening of his stay the wine waiter came for his order. He asked for a bottle of ginger ale; the waiter returned to tell him they had none but they had bitter ale. He asked if that was

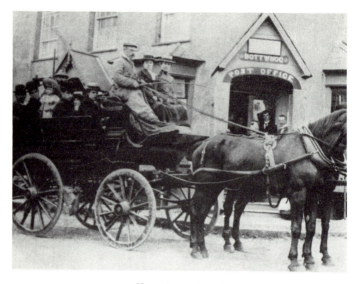

Horse bus and mail

alcoholic and was told, "Not really." For a week he enjoyed his drink of bitter ale at dinner and his appetite improved. When he returned home he felt much better and told the story to his wife. She exclaimed, with deep feeling, "But my dear that is ordinary beer — that dreadful alcoholic drink, beer." We have no record of what followed; I believe he was a deacon too!

When we arrived in 1925, the hostelries still catered for the farming and country people with their horses and traps, although by now there were a few cars. These were looked after by several garages that had suddenly appeared, and they also gave service to the cyclist and to the few motor cyclists of the district.

Buses were to be seen in much greater numbers than in my school days, and were gradually squeezing out the old horse drawn coaches that had served the principle villages in the surrounding area. In fact some of the coach owners had become private bus companies and gave a very good cheap service to the people, and often carried the mail. There was ample space for parking in the Station Square where there were also a few private motor taxicabs for hire.

The private development of the west end of the shore had started in 1890. A row of ugly terraced houses had been built, three stories high, many of which were now boarding houses. The tenants of these houses depended for their living on summer visitors. The beach and its attractions were very popular; there were many holiday visitors and the landladies' business was thriving. At the back of these houses a recreation field had been made in 1893. It had a good cycling track that had been much used in the past for cycle racing, but was not used much at the present time. The field itself was now a football field in the winter and used for tennis and sports meetings in the summer. This was a great asset to the town and attracted many visitors. In 1911 Gustav Hamel, an early pioneer of flying, visited the town with his aeroplane. He thought there was enough room for him to take off from this ground, but alas it happened otherwise, and he touched the stone wall at the end of the field when beginning to ascend and crashed. So the demonstration was a failure but the pilot was unhurt.

There were horse trams owned by the same developer and these ran to Llanbedrog three miles away. They started in the centre of the town and ran on tracks to the beaches and thence along the shore. They were especially useful to the town folk and visitors in providing transport from the town to both the south and west ends of the shore.

When evening dances were held at the Hall in an old mansion at Llanbedrog, parties of young people journeyed there by these horse trams. The trip there and back was all part of the evening's enjoyment, especially as so often happened mischievous young men would jump from the tram and run to the next points to switch them over before the horses got there, in order to derail the tram and delay the journey home. There are many of the older generation who can remember with delight those summer evenings and the journeys on the old horse trams.

These trams had open sides and no roof and were known locally as 'toast racks'. The local ones that ran from the town to the beach had sides in case of accident to the children, and were later fitted with a cover against the weather. They were quite an institution, and often during my life in England I came across people whose only recollection of Pwllheli was the 'Toast Rack'! They only ceased to run after a bad storm and high tide had damaged the track so badly in the winter of 1931.

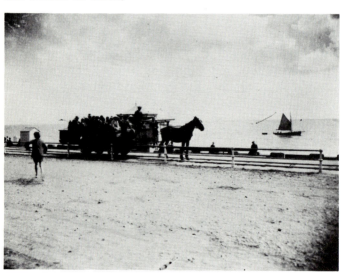

Horse tram

Early in the century an inner harbour had been developed at great expense. This reclamation from the sea made it possible to extend the railway into the centre of the town for passenger traffic. The old station half a mile away was used afterwards as a goods railway yard. This change had been a great improvement and much appreciated by those who depended on the terminus for all journeys outside the area. There had been high hopes that the harbour and small island in its centre would benefit the town financially but alas this was not so. In order to raise the level of the water in the harbour which had two rivers running into it a wall had been built near the lock gates. The result was catastrophic because this caused flooding along the courses of both rivers. The idea was therefore abandoned and the lock gates left open permanently. In time the wall disappeared and there followed severe silting in the harbour itself. Owing to the expense, the harbour could not be dredged satisfactorily. The final result was that the coastal traders had to dock in the outer harbour and their goods, coal and other merchandise brought to the quayside by lighters drawn by a small tug. The lighters were still using the harbour in 1925.

Sea fishing was carried on from Pwllheli at this time and a well-known person, Miss Rebecca Clarke owned several fishing boats. She kept a shop in the centre of the town and sold fruit, vegetables, game and fish. We could always depend on getting fresh fish from her shop. Miss Clarke was certainly one of the great personalities of the town both before this time and for many years to come. She employed local men as crews for her fishing boats, some of whom were descendants of the crews of Fleetwood trawlers that had fished in Cardigan Bay and afterwards chosen to settle down in South Caernarfonshire. The fishing boats used to bring home good catches of plaice, sole, herring, and mackerel, when in season. Miss Clarke had been born in the town not far from her shop; her father was an immigrant from Yorkshire and her mother was a local Welsh woman. Miss Clarke was a most successful business woman as well as a good employer and popular with her customers. It may be that her kindness to the poor, often unknown to the public and her keen sense of humour contributed to her popularity. There was a very good instance of the latter when a wealthy, titled bachelor landowner called at her shop as was his custom when in the town and said, "Good morning, Miss Clarke — when are you getting married?" From behind the counter she curtsied and replied, "Just name the date, Sir."

Miss Clarke was not the only prominent woman in the business life of the town. There were others and perhaps one of the outstanding personalities was Mrs Thomas (who later became Mrs Griffith). She was the daughter of a manse in South Wales and after her marriage settled down in Pwllheli and established a small cafe called The Gwalia. This developed into an extensive restaurant, and it became quite a social centre in the town where folks could enjoy a chat with friends while having lunch or tea, and it was always packed to overflowing on market days. She never forgot that she was the daughter of the manse, and was proud of the fact that during her fifty years in the restaurant she never accepted any money for food or service from 'the Cloth'. Mrs Thomas was not only an excellent cook but showed great artistry in cake-making and her pastries and cakes were always in great demand. In spite of her busy life managing her establishment, she found time to demonstrate and lecture to various women's meetings such as Women's Institutes around the country. She also brought up a family of three — two daughters, and a son who is now a Canon of the Church.

In 1835 a private gas company had been formed and had supplied the town with gas for street lighting and public buildings. When we arrived in 1925 we found the streets still lit by gas and many homes were supplied with gas for lighting and cooking, although candles and paraffin lamps were still used in many houses.

It took us a little while to get used to the narrow streets of the town after the wider streets of the bigger cities, and the tall buildings in England. Indeed, on market day, the crowded High Street was almost like our conception of a modern pedestrian precinct, except for the occasional car that slowly ploughed its way through. The small shops were mostly family businesses, and I was surprised to find that so many of them were exactly as I had remembered them from my schoolboy days. The only change was that in some instances the son and not the father was now behind the counter and in charge of the business. The shopkeepers were all very proud of the service they gave to the town, and it was a friendly and efficient shopping centre.

In 1925 electric power was just arriving from the North Wales Power Company, and we were fortunate in having it installed in our new home at Brynhyfryd before the end of that year. It was a cheap and efficient service. Later, after we had left, it was taken over by the Merseyside and North Wales Electricity Board.

The fire service in those days was very primitive and manned entirely by volunteers. It was only after one of the bigger Chapels had been burned down by a fire-raiser that the service was modernised.

There was an interesting story told of a fire that occurred some time after we had left when the South Beach Hotel caught fire. It happened one Sunday afternoon and a servant girl was sent to tell the captain of the fire brigade. He happened to be the Superintendent of the Sunday School in the centre of the town and was talking to the members at the time.

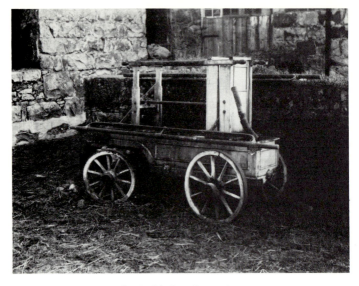

Pwllheli's first fire engine

The girl waited in the porch for him to finish his address and give the blessing — by the time they arrived with the appliances the hotel had been completely gutted!

There were several Chapels of different denominations and one Church in the town. They were all well attended and had great influence on the life of the people. Perhaps this was due to the aftermath of the religious revival that had taken place at the beginning of the century, although this was only remembered by the older folk. The religious bodies succeeded in attracting many young people by organising social functions, especially concerts and singing meetings.

There were two political clubs, Liberal and Conservative, but these were not very well supported and had little influence at this time. Pwllheli had never lacked men and women who were willing and able to give their time and knowledge for the welfare of the town without political motives or bias.

Cornelius Roberts, a butcher by trade, was one such personality who played a very important part in the life of Pwllheli during the first fifty years or more of this century. He was mayor of the town several times, a Justice of the Peace, an Alderman of the County, and a Deacon at one of the principle Calvinist Chapels in the town. He also took a great interest in the work of the Sunday School and helped to found a special Children's Sunday School in the poorer part of the town. His outspoken views were not always well received, but he was an able debater who could argue convincingly and insisted on being heard. In the Chapel this sometimes brought him into conflict with the Minister, Morgan Griffith who was also a man with strong views, and there were then harsh words spoken. It is just as well that it did not reach the fisticuffs stage for they were both fit and strong, and it would have been a heavyweight contest! As well as his other activities he was captain of the voluntary fire brigade, and also encouraged the work of the Salvation Army.

My earliest recollections of him were seeing him at the Agricultural Showground displaying his light horses and driving his gig, and often winning prizes. He also showed cattle and other livestock, for he had a farm within the boundary of the town. I was very interested in hearing from him about a visit he had made to the United States when he was a young man. He visited the Indian Settlements and felt that these American Indians were being unfairly treated by the United States Government, for, he argued, their land had been taken from them and they were the original inhabitants of the country. He succeeded in obtaining an audience with the President and was very outspoken to everyone in authority that he met. But all to no avail. As a Welshman he had great sympathy for these

American Indians, for he felt that his own country had been similarly treated. This was Welsh Nationalism seventy years ago.

The development of Pwllheli into a beautiful seaside resort was very much in his mind in later years. When I met him on my visits to the town from Bristol, he used to discuss with me the possibility of refuse-tipping along the banks of the river, so as to provide pleasant riverside walks from the town, and create a park on its outskirts. That was one of his visions, and I encouraged him as much as possible by pointing out that refuse-tipping could be carried out quite near inhabited areas without being a nuisance if it was done scientifically. I suggested that he could see how this had been done successfully in larger towns in England. All this happened over forty years ago.

He had been a great friend of my father all his life, for he was brought up in a little hamlet near my great-grandfather's home at Clogwyn where my father had spent much of his youth. He went to see my father when he was dying at the age of eighty four, and when I saw my father shortly afterwards he said how Cornelius had worried him because he had insisted that my father was six months older than he was. Father was equally insistent that the opposite was true. Statistically six months in eighty four years is not significant, but I suppose when one is that age six months matters a great deal.

Education

There was only one change in the educational pattern in the town since my early days. This was the appearance of a large Central School. The Infants School was the same, and so was the Elementary School, but one Church School had been closed. The County School which had been founded in 1903 continued to flourish. At one time Pwllheli did have an opportunity of becoming an educational centre. A gift of £1,000 was made in the seventeenth century to build an endowed school for free education. Pwllheli was selected as the best centre for the three counties, and the school existed for about 150 years. However, the Treasurer of the School borrowed £800 of the capital for his personal use at a nominal interest rate. What finally happened to this money and to the school is not recorded.

Education was a problem for the parents of both middle and working class families. There was no money to spare in either case, and when a child from any of these homes showed promise at school it was the wish of the parents to see him or her achieving academic success. This could be attributed to two desires — one for education and knowledge, and the other in order that the child could enter a profession such as medicine, law or the church. Their motto was, "We want to see our children having a better chance in life than we had."

The University College at Aberystwyth had been established through the contributions of ordinary people in Wales, in their keen desire to get a higher education for their children.

An example of how much some parents were prepared to sacrifice to see their children educated as they wished was the story of one of my fellow students at the County School. He wanted to enter the Church but he was not content with finding the easiest way to do so. He was determined to obtain higher education and to understand the fundamental issues involved in its practice. As boys of that age do, we looked lightly upon his attitude but we much admired some of his qualities. He had entered school with a scholarship which gave him free tuition only. He had so far passed all his examinations but not with outstanding success, for he did not pretend to be a bright boy and had considerable difficulty with some subjects such as mathematics. However, he had patience and perseverance, which is what is best described as grit, and a mental persistence in trying to understand whatever he might be studying. I understand now what excellent qualities these were — Charles Dickens said that a genius is a person with an infinite capacity for taking pains. After reaching matriculation standard at the County School he sat for a scholarship to Aberystwyth and won one for £30 a year. With this came more problems. His widowed mother owned a terraced house which she had bought after working hard to earn her livelihood and living sparingly. At once she sold her house, and with the money took rooms in Aberystwyth where she could look after her son. He did well, obtained a scholarship to Oxford and here won the Greek prize of the University. He ended his career as the Principal of a Theological College. What an invincible team the two made in their struggle, and what an example to so many parents today who are not prepared to let their children stay in school because their earnings are required to swell the family exchequer. This story which is only an example of many similar ones ended rather sadly. At the age of retirement he died. He was unable to sit and enjoy his memories of struggles, of ups and downs, of victories and of a wonderful little mother. Could it be that he burnt the candle down to the end of the wick?

Changes in Countryside and Country Life

As I drove out on visits to patients in the countryside the first great change I noticed was that the main roads were now tarmacadamed. I remember how as children we had laughed at an elderly son of a nearby farmer who had returned home after spending many years in South Wales and the West of England, and had described vividly how the main roads had been covered with tar to stop the dust, with great success. My mother was horrified at the idea that we should be bringing tar into the house on our boots. And now, after twenty five years, the main roads were almost free of dust. Public pressure had been brought to bear to insist on this amenity because the traps, bicycles, motor cycles and cars now had rubber tyres. The by-roads had not been treated, but this did not matter to such an extent, as they were used mostly by

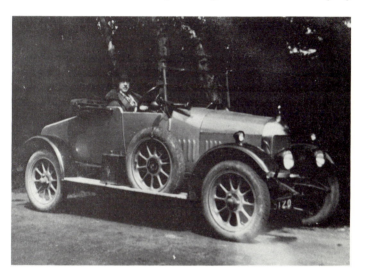

Joan in practice days

farm vehicles and there was very little traffic except on market days. On our journeys we often met sheep, cattle and horses grazing along the roadside, but we were never afraid of meeting cars being driven in haste for there was all the time in the world, and nobody had been bitten by the 'speed bug'.

Here I must pay tribute to the bull-nosed Morris Cowleys that I have already mentioned. They required very little maintenance and the total cost of each was about £100 (licence and insurance included). They served us well for over three years.

The countryside had changed very little since my boyhood days. Most of the old, familiar landmarks were still to be seen, but it was sad that some of the privately owned forests had been cut down. They had not been completely cleared because only those trees useful for timber had been cut down, as had some of the finer trees from the small coppices. I suppose this was only to be expected, for there had been a great demand for timber during the World War when supplies to this island had been cut off. Unfortunately no planting seemed to have occurred to replace this loss, although the war had been over for more than six years.

The slopes of Yr Eifl near my old home had always been bare of trees, and the only shelter for the animals had been the stone walls. What a difference a few clumps of trees would have made to the shelter of both animals and ourselves from the wintry blasts.

There did not seem to have been much recent building of houses in the town or villages. A few new ones had been built on the outskirts for middle class families, and a sprinkling of council houses for the workers in various parts of the Peninsula.

However, what saddened me most of all was to see the War Memorials in nearly every village, some were just plaques and others statues, but all with their lists of local boys who had died in the Great War of 1914-1918. The local battalions had been in the thick of the fighting, and many of these village communities had suffered severe losses; there was hardly a family which had not been affected, and in Nefyn many had lost some one at sea, for this was the home of many officers and seamen serving in the Merchant Navy. Two local lads had been killed whilst serving in the Flying Corps at a time when flying was in its infancy. I wondered what the attitude of the people would be to all these tragedies. Would they raise their voices and say "never again"? Their attitude was very different. They were distressed that so many young lives had been sacrificed and blamed the politicians all over the world who, they thought, were playing their own game and getting something out of it. They felt that life was so short and they wanted to forget. This was the kind of sound then that came from the 'silent majority'.

Many of the old Welsh country cottages were falling into decay. Many were still occupied, but was it my fancy that the little gardens were not as spick and span as they used to be? Some that we visited were occupied by elderly couples or widows who were not capable of doing the work themselves, and whose young folk had left the village to look for work away from their old homes. I had the impression that many of the younger men were not prepared to work round the clock as their fathers had done. They had returned after fighting for their country and had looked forward to being able to obtain work in the country they had defended. One had much sympathy with them but nevertheless realised that it was the homes that were suffering.

In a practice so widespread we became acquainted with the home conditions of rich and poor, town and country folk, young and old. The anxiety of some parents to give their children a better opportunity through education than they had themselves has already been mentioned. Even so, only a small minority of the young folk were given this chance. On leaving school the village girl from a working class home often went into domestic service, especially if she was one of several children. The mother was often glad to have one daughter at home to help her, but was happy to see another given a good home either on a farm or in the town. The wages were low, but in the majority of cases the compensation of living in a comfortable home, well fed and with a room of her own was not to be despised. Unless they left to get married many of these girls settled down, and we often visited farms where a girl had been a help for many years and was looked upon as one of the family.

Although there was some improvement in housing conditions taking place, the housework was still laborious especially on the farms where the farmer's wife was glad of extra help. Washing day meant hours of work — water to be heated on the fire or in a copper, often in an outhouse; the kitchen range was usually the only means of cooking and supplying hot water. About this time some of the villages were being connected to a main water supply, but most of the small cottages and the farms still had to rely on the well or pump and had only outdoor sanitation.

The only two professions for the more intelligent and ambitious girls were nursing and teaching. In the town there were more jobs as shop assistants or office clerks for those parents who could not afford the expense of their training or wanted their daughters to stay at home. The boys had more choice than the girls. They could become apprenticed to builders or plumbers, train as motor mechanics in a local garage or learn to drive a tradesman's van or a bus, for these were becoming more numerous. The majority of the lads from the farms or the villages returned after leaving school to help their parents or become employed on the land. The big cities like London, Manchester or even Liverpool seemed a long way off, and to take a job so far away was a big undertaking for most young people.

Farming seemed to have been changing in several ways. In my attempt to look back a few years to find a yardstick on which to measure these changes I was fortunate in having an old friend, Glynne Jones M.B.E. who has recently retired after being employed by the Ministry of Agriculture as Livestock Officer for thirty one years. Born and brought up on a farm of 360 acres, Neigwl Plas, he lent me his father's old diary which gave me a detailed account of all the wages paid by him at Neigwl Plas since 1868 until his death from an accident in 1920 at the age of 81. In 1900, when I was a youngster, he employed ten workers, including two women whose wages were half that of a man. The wages bill for six months for all ten workers was £90 and for the whole year it amounted to £170, and board and lodgings. The winter wages were less than the summer ones; he used to employ a few part-time helpers for special occasions. It was interesting to note that thirteen years later, at the beginning of the First World War, the bailiff's wages had risen to £14.10.0. a half year. This was an increase of ten shillings for six months in a period of thirteen years. The staff at that time was fewer by one woman, so the wages bill remained about the same.

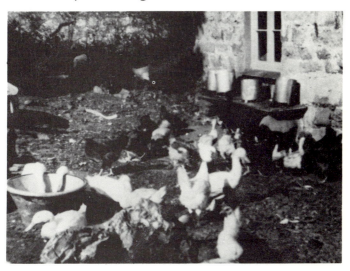

Old time farm yard

In 1918 the Agricultural Wages Board had come into existence and his wages bill had jumped to £155 for the half year. The bailiff was now paid £31 for six months; the staff was then reduced to six men and one woman. By 1926, seven years after the end of the war the wages of the bailiff were down to £28.10.0. a half year. This reduction in staff and decrease in pay was for a wholly economic cause and not due to mechanisation of the land which was only just beginning. The number of farm workers was limited during the war although agricultural workers were exempt from military service. Prices of farm produce had risen during the war and no doubt this fact was taken into consideration by the Wages Board. When farming relapsed again later the wages and the employment of labour both declined.

During the period mentioned it is of interest to record the prices received by farmers for their stock. Before the war, a good milking cow could be bought for £12 to £14, a calf for 25/-, a sheep for £2.10.0. and a fat pig for £4. As the result of the war, prices more than doubled and farmers were paying no income tax. They were therefore able to put a little money aside and this helped them to weather the post-war depression when prices dropped once again to their pre-war level.

During the post-war period, therefore, we could not expect much change in farming because the farmers had no incentive to bring in new methods. The tractor had appeared on the larger farms and as a result more work was done and much time saved. Ploughing in particular with the multi-furrow plough cut the time to a quarter, and at the same time reduced the amount of labour and of horses with which to do the work. In the same way the baler made the hay harvest less of a toil as did also the binder in the corn harvest. Great changes were on the way but had not reached the smaller farms which were the majority in our part,

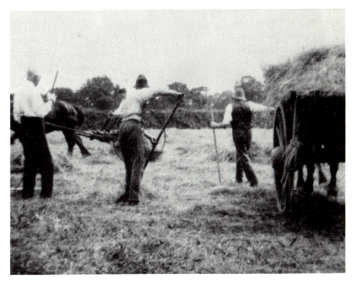

Hay harvest

where it was not an economic proposition to acquire the equipment, although some employed a contractor for the harvesting or other jobs requiring mechanical aids if and when they could find one.

The days had passed when women were hired to follow the scythe or mower to bundle the hay or stook the corn, but these arduous tasks performed by their mothers are recalled by some children, and may even be within living memory of a few old village women.

A prominent feature of the agricultural scene in these parts during my childhood days had been the Agricultural shows at Pwllheli in the summer and at Nefyn at Easter. The horse sections — heavy and light — were very well patronised and were fine displays. There were cattle, sheep, poultry sections and also a dog show. At Pwllheli a large tent was allotted to the display of farm produce, and there used to be keen competition among farmers' wives who competed for prizes in butter, cheese, and jams, as well as cakes and bread. These shows were very popular with the farmers and their families and the meetings formed a rallying point for social gatherings to which they looked forward from one year to the next. These shows had not changed much in their character in the last twenty years but the number of entries in the livestock sections was smaller. I imagine that this was probably due to the labour of preparing for the occasion with fewer helpers. This may have discouraged many would-be competitors. The reduction in the number of entries made the task of the organisers more difficult.

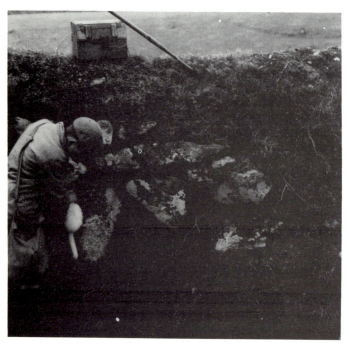

Ferreting

Although food had been short during the war and large numbers of rabbits had been killed for human consumption, it was very apparent as we travelled about the countryside that they were still a pest. The damage done to farm crops was inestimable, and the return that came from selling them for food did not nearly compensate for the loss by the damage they did to the crops. Here and there efforts were being made, but where there was poor agricultural land no attempt at all had been made to eradicate them. It was very apparent to anyone who gave the problem a moment's thought that a combined effort was required if all the land was to be freed from this pest.

In my boyhood days ferreting was a popular sport and helped to decrease the rabbit population. There was a very deaf old man who used to visit our farm with his ferrets and I enjoyed many hours watching him at work. First he examined 'the earth', as he called it, counting the entrances and exits. He then blocked up some of the holes with stones and turf and netted others through which he thought the rabbits might escape. Then he let the ferret into a hole on the other side of the hedge and knelt down at another hole with his ear to the wire netting. More than once, owing to his deafness, he was completely unaware of a rabbit breathing down his ear trying to escape!

General Practice

We found a considerable amount of ill health amongst people of all classes, and there were many reasons that we felt could account for this. There was an underlying economic worry amongst the farmers; most of them were tenants and did not own their farms and they therefore lacked security. After the flourishing days of the war a depression of farm prices followed, and although labour was cheap there was a vicious circle resulting in a fall in productivity and in farming income. Superimposed on this tension was a lack of certain factors in the diet and a probable excess of tea drinking. Lack of personal hygiene and comfortable conditions in the home, especially during the winter led to much ill health. It was very easy to give good advice on all these matters, but a doctor must be practical and try to fit the advice to the ability of the patient to follow it.

Always it seems in medicine that 'the New' appears more attractive than the old, and with the advance of science there is always a preference for modern treatments, rather than the proven with their success based on experience. This would account for some of the catastrophies of recent years, and naturally there are probably more that have not been exposed to the light of day because they have been individual or small in number. All practising doctors have great responsibilities whether they be general practitioners or hospital specialists. The family doctor is nearer to his patient and so both his mistakes and his successes remain with him, to torment or cheer him as the case may be.

Amongst the working class this condition of tension already described existed even to a greater degree than amongst the farmers. There was little security for the family, although the recent Insurance Act had done something to help the worker with sickness benefit and a medical service. Yet no state medical scheme existed to help members of the family who were more likely to fall ill and to need medical care, than the father. Sickness therefore meant that they had to seek medical help and that meant an expense they could ill afford, and which was a drain on the small family exchequer. As might be expected, therefore, the cost was a deterrent to seeking early advice and often resulted in the sufferer getting worse and prolonging the illness, possibly resulting in a permanent crippling condition. I often look back with amazement that after more than nineteen hundred years of Christianity so little had been done in a so-called enlightened country to deal with such contingencies. It is no good blaming the Government of the day, for even nowadays there is a fatalistic attitude, not necessarily associated with ignorance, of "it cannot happen to me" towards accidents, cancer through smoking and other diseases. Surely training even more than education is required to guard against the dangers to health.

My attitude to the prevention of disease is indicated by the following story. A deputation of leading Spanish civil servants came to Bristol some years ago to study local government. They were brought to my office with an interpreter and the first remark made was, "You are the person, doctor, who tells us not to do what we want to do; is that not what preventive medicine means?" I explained that I took a different view altogether, and that as Professor of Preventive Medicine it was my duty to spread knowledge concerning dangers to health, and how to keep healthy. Man has a free will and can use that knowledge or not as he wishes.

We, in our own small way tried to help the poorer families in and around the town. Sooner or later they were compelled to come and seek our help even though they could seldom meet our costs, much less give us a profit. But what was even more distressing was that many of the parents were deterred from coming to seek assistance because they knew they were not in a position to pay, and did not want to receive charity. They waited to see what nature and a little home treatment would do before coming for help and this often made our task much harder. An insurance collector in the town approached me with a suggestion that he should form a club to which the families of the men who were on our 'panels' could contribute six-pence a week, and we would be responsible for treating them and supplying medicines for all the family who fell ill. More than a hundred families joined this club and we were able to call at their homes and give an occasional word of advice before illness occurred.

There is much to be said for social security. Where there exists a happy family life, such security can add still more to the happiness of the home, and its absence can produce the opposite effect. Many parents were so concerned with the future that they were unable to enjoy the present, and the resulting anxiety reduced their vitality and adversely affected the atmosphere of the home. On the other hand too much security can be disastrous to a certain type of person. Norman Collins in his account of Dr Johnson concludes, "a mind like Dr Johnson's is rare, but sloth such as Dr Johnson's is common and Johnson was an author who worked with zest only when the bailiffs of fate were greedily pressing for an early settlement of accounts ...".

The traders in the town were not affected to such a marked degree as the farmers by the slump following the war, but the briskness of their trade depended on the standard of living of the working class and the financial state of the farmers. Their bad debt problems became worse when there was not much money about.

During the years in which we practised, the family doctor held a closer relationship with his patient than any other social worker including the minister, the parson or the lawyer. Even so, at times he would realise that there was an underlying worry undivulged which could retard recovery. People varied very much in the ease with which they unburdened their secret worries, but they knew full well that these secrets were safe in a doctor's repository, and most acted accordingly. Thus the doctor was often loaded with added responsibilities which were only indirectly associated with his patient's health, and the advice he had to give gave rise to much anxious thinking.

We all differ in the way we suffer pain and sickness and in the way we respond to treatment. It is because of this more than anything else that there should be continuity of treatment by the same doctor. Of course there should be consultation when diagnosis is in doubt. I myself found a second opinion from my wife or our colleague, Dr Jack Lewis, most valuable as no doubt they did with me. When the group of doctors is small the patient gets the best of both worlds. I belonged to the old school which laid great stress on the bedside manner. My teachers at the Middlesex Hospital taught us the importance of 'serving' scientific medicine to the patient in the most attractive way possible. In those days I knew many doctors who paid more attention to the 'service' than to the 'goods' they delivered but all the same the patient always seemed to be most satisfied. The ideal, of course, is to give both the 'service' and the 'goods' equally well.

The mind has a very great effect on the body and its ability to recover from diseases. I had many examples of this when dealing with patients. One young woman, a gentle refined little lady had married the wrong man for her — a rough, uncouth type. After fighting the good fight for some years she took to her bed. Her family knew part of her trouble and moved her to live with her sister. I was called to attend her but neither Joan nor I could find anything physically the matter with her. She would not eat, until she became so weak that she could not take any food. Her sister told me that she just wanted to die and I could do nothing to help. We considered various forms of treatment and even removing her to hospital, but all suggestions were rejected. She died.

Another middle-aged lady was seriously ill with pneumonia — in pre-antibiotic days. She was delirious when I saw her first and remained seriously ill for

some days. She was not a physically strong person,
but I was fortunate in finding a relative who was a
trained nurse to come and nurse her for a couple of
weeks. She recovered. Later she told me that when
she had lucid intervals in her delirium she had wanted
to tell me that she was not going to die. She felt that
she had not finished her task of bringing up the family
and was most determined to stay alive.

Tuberculosis was common in young adolescents in
those days. Some of the patients I had to treat were
unforgettable because they and their families refused
sanatorium treatment. Sanatoria for these tubercular
cases had been in existence since the Act of 1911.
Cases of infectious tuberculosis should never be
nursed at home, but too often the sanatoria were far
away and the patients, particularly if they had
comfortable homes, refused to leave them. This
attitude created a grave risk to the healthy members
of the family and I saw more than one calamity that
resulted.

There was the case of a young girl, aged seventeen,
living in the town with the appearance described by
Hippocrates over two thousand years ago — pink face,
delicate skin, blue eyes and shoulder blades "having
the appearance of wings". She would only stay in bed
when she was too tired to get up. I failed to persuade
her to go to a sanatorium. She died after a short
illness of acute lung tuberculosis.

Another case was that of a young lorry driver. I
was summoned to see him when he fell ill with what
he described as bronchitis. His sputum was full of
tubercle germs and I did my best to persuade him to
go to a sanatorium. He had a good little home, a wife
who was very capable and a small boy nearly two
years old. Even with the help of the Tuberculosis
Officer and warnings of the danger to the child we
failed to get him to hospital. Within a matter of
weeks the child died of tubercular meningitis. The

father was heart-broken and died soon afterwards.

There was also the danger that a girl suffering from quiescent tuberculosis of the lung could become a maid in a home where there were young children, or a teacher in a school. When such a case deteriorated and was later discovered it resulted in a very unpleasant problem for the medical adviser. Considerable pressure was often applied by the patient to prevent the condition from being divulged, especially if the person did not have severe symptoms but was nevertheless infectious. To maintain secrecy regarding his patient's condition and at the same time take steps to prevent the risk of infection to others is always a real dilemma, requiring tact and courage on the part of the doctor.

But I would not like my readers to think that a country doctor's life was all sadness. There was much to cheer him and brighten his days. One day I was called to see an old farmer who had earache. Apparently he had been getting more and more deaf in the last few years. I examined him and found his ears completely blocked with hard wax so I gave him some ear drops to soften this and returned a few days later to syringe his ears. In order to do this I sat him on a chair in the little courtyard where there was a better light. I cleared one ear and he jumped up amazed that he could hear sounds around him that he had not heard for years and he was thrilled. Whilst this was happening his bailiff went by and heard him. He called me urgently and whispered, "For heaven's sake doctor, don't clear his other ear, he hears too much as it is!"

Although, when we arrived, many of the old characters had departed others were coming along to fill the gaps. I was delighted to meet again some that still were alive and to renew old friendships. I met one such old man on a Saturday afternoon on my way out of town to visit a patient. He was Bob Thomas, a roadmender from near my old home who had always had a cheerful word to say to everyone who passed by. I used to think that he did as much to maintain the morale of the local people as he did to improve the road. On Saturday afternoons he used to be seen tramping along the main road, a distance of about three miles from his home, to get a drink at his nearest pub in Pwllheli. He was nearing the town when I saw him and I stopped the car and called to him. He at once crossed the road and I asked him if he would like to accompany me to Llithfaen where my patient was living. "Certainly," said he, and jumped in beside me. I then reminded him of an occasion when I was a boy at a singing festival in the big Chapel at Llithfaen and he had been sitting in the front row of the gallery. He was a fine singer and very proud of his voice. I reminded him of the hymn sung on that occasion and he at once agreed with me and started singing it at the top of his voice. There was not much traffic about and those who were walking or driving along the road stopped to listen to the voice coming from the little open two-seater car. We had to pass the 'bush telephone', the old tailors and their friends leaning on the stone wall at Ty'nlon, and as we turned the corner opposite their house Bob Thomas closed his eyes and sang with even greater gusto. I could imagine the little audience saying, "Poor old Bob — and so early in the day. We've never seen him drunk before. Why should the doctor be taking him home?" They must have been still more confounded when half an hour later we returned and Bob still singing. When visiting the district some years later I called to see him on his death bed. It was then my turn to say a cheerful word to him.

Another story about hymn singing concerns a man from our village called William John Williams. He was well known as a musician of considerable merit. Indeed with a little more ambition and energy he could have reached a much higher level in the musical world. But he was a quiet, modest man not given to broadcasting his views, although what he said was always worth listening to. His father had composed one of the finest hymn tunes in the Welsh Calvinistic hymnal under the title of 'Pwllheli'. One day a music teacher approached William John and asked him if he would compose music for a hymn which he could use at a concert. He obligingly bestirred himself and produced the music. A few months later he was at a local Eisteddfod and listened to an adjudicator paying a glowing tribute to the winner of a hymn tune, and the adjudicator was so impressed with it that he went and played it on the piano. William John turned to his friend and said, "I think I know that tune." He was able to confirm this when the winner stepped up to receive the prize. It was the tune he had composed for him. No action was taken! The last time I had a long chat with him was when he accompanied me in the car for a long distance visit to see a patient north of Nefyn. As we were passing a churchyard he asked me to stop. He then pointed to a high stone wall facing along one side of the graveyard. In his slow, carefully phrased words he told me that an old sea captain had wished to be buried against the wall, standing up and facing east. It had involved a long dig down to cover the coffin standing on end. William John's final comment was, "I'm afraid the poor devil has been on his backside for many years by now."

> The best-laid schemes o' mice an' men
> Gang aft a-gley,
>
> *R. Burns*

* * * * *

One of my patients was an elderly business man with no family and plenty of this world's goods. He was very ill and struggled well in his fight against a serious disease concerning which he had sought the advice of many specialists. Finally he decided to leave himself in my hands. When he died I was informed that it was his wish that a vein in his body should be cut to make sure he was not buried alive. The ceremony was arranged and his executor was present as directed in the will. When it was over and everyone was satisfied that the circulation of the blood had ceased and he had really died, the executor remarked that I was now entitled to a fee. He had directed that I be asked to perform the operation but not to be paid unless everyone was satisfied he was really dead! I could well imagine his words, "Don't pay the little d... unless he carries out my wishes...."

Saturday afternoon was always a busy time. The country people used to come to town by bus to do their shopping, and left it till the last minute to call on us for their medicines before their bus was due to leave for home. This usually meant a hectic hour for us before six o'clock. On one such occasion I blotted my copy book! A well known tenor whose bardic name was 'Tenorydd yr Eifl' came to pay a small account. We started talking about his singing and in no time he was singing to me at the top of his voice one of his favourite songs. Joan came to investigate and found a waiting crowd listening as near to the consulting room door as they could get. I wonder how many I caused to miss their last bus!

Dr J. Gwenogfryn Evans was a distinguished Oxford scholar and an Honorary Graduate of that University where he had made some notable contributions by his research work. He had achieved this high standing in the academic world by hard work and in difficult circumstances. It was my privilege to be his medical attendant for three years. He lived in retirement at Llanbedrog where he built a large stone house with a library modelled on some corner of the Bodleian

Library at Oxford that he had in mind. I spent many happy hours with him, listening to his experiences and his words of wisdom. We had an arrangement whereby if I was shown into his study with my hat in my hand and wearing an overcoat it was a social call as a friend, but if I had left my hat and coat in the hall it meant work and I was his physician on duty. He was never afraid of speaking his mind, and I well remember a reprimand he gave to an English country gentleman who had settled down in these parts and who, as was the custom, had been made a Justice of the Peace. This gentleman had complained that Welsh was spoken in court. Dr Gwenogfryn was himself a J.P. and he wrote to the papers to express his view that no one should be allowed to sit in judgment on a case in Wales unless he understood the language of the accused person. It is only now that such outspoken comments are to be heard. In those days it was an unusual and courageous outburst. He died two years after we left and was buried in a grave beside his wife, in a part of the rocky hillside of his own garden which had been specially consecrated for this purpose.

Joan's Impressions

The following is an account that Joan wrote of some of her impressions and memories of the years she practised in Wales.

I had very little knowledge of Wales and the Welsh people before coming to live and work in Pwllheli. Like many English people my conception of the country was of beautiful scenery in the north and coalmines in the south — a land of poets and singers with a language as little used as Latin. But when I did settle down in Caernarfonshire I was soon to have these old ideas shattered.

To begin with I found that the Welsh language was

very much alive. The younger folk were mostly
bilingual, but Welsh was the language used in the
family circle and many of the older generation could
not understand English; some who could were often
shy of speaking to me in English even though they
might possibly understand what I said. Even when the
children left home to take jobs or go to college their
letters were usually written in Welsh.

My first experience in trying to deal with the
language problem came soon after we started
practising. Being market day it was a busy afternoon
in the surgery and a call came to visit an old lady in
a near-by village. My husband was too busy to leave
and, knowing the old lady could not speak English, he
gave me a quick lesson in the Welsh words for parts
of the body. I had picked up one or two phrases and
by using the right inflection to indicate a question or
affirmation I was able to examine her and arrive at a
diagnosis. On my return my husband wanted to know
how I had fared. I told him that I had diagnosed her
trouble but that I hadn't understood much of what she
had tried to tell me. There was one word that often
cropped up — 'brenin mawr' — and when I asked
what part of the body it was my husband laughed. It
was a mild swear word meaning 'Good Heavens'.

Although there were many women doctors already
in practice I was the first to arrive in these parts and
expected to find some prejudice in the attitude towards
a woman doctor. My first midwifery case confirmed
my fears! There were few telephones in this area and
the husband had cycled three miles to call their doctor
and had found that he was not available. He then came
to us and asked if I would come and attend his wife.
He gave me directions to reach the isolated farmhouse
on the side of the mountain. After leaving the car at
the foot of the hill and taking the winding path up to
the house I found the wife already in labour. She was
being attended by a 'Mother Gamp' whose surprise at

seeing me, a woman doctor who could not speak Welsh, instead of their usual family practitioner was understandable. She left me to cope with a rather distressed patient, but the family were very helpful. The case ended happily and the mother and baby did well. From then on I found no prejudice in spite of being a 'foreigner'!

I soon realised that the person who led the most exacting and strenuous life in the community was the district nurse midwife. She was always on duty and had a district of several square miles with a very scattered population. Her only means of transport was her bicycle, and even this was useless on many of her visits to cottages and farms on the steep hillsides. I learnt later that her salary at that time was only twenty five shillings a week and out of that she had to pay for her lodgings, ten shillings a week, and supply her own uniform. She equipped her bag with dressings etc. obtained from the local chemist who was paid for the goods by the County Authority. Any money she received from patients had to be paid over to the Council. She had very little free time and often had to go on her round after being up all night. Officially she was supposed to have one half day a week free, but if there was much illness around she had to forego this time off. Many years later I met one of these nurses and asked her if she had enjoyed her time as a district midwife. She replied that she had been really happy and that her work had been so rewarding (and she certainly did not mean financially!).

I looked after most of the maternity cases and sick babies in the practice. I soon realised that attending these cases in an isolated country community was very different from my experience in a London hospital where every assistance was forthcoming. Our nearest hospital, apart from the poor law institution, was twenty five miles away and no adequate ambulance service was available. Fortunately the majority of cases were uncomplicated. It was difficult to persuade mothers to come and consult us during pregnancy, which meant that I was often only called in at the last minute. There were probably two reasons for this — firstly the expense of visits to the surgery or of the doctor's visit to the home, and secondly a lack of appreciation of the importance of medical care during pregnancy for the sake of both mother and baby. It was difficult to carry out strict hygiene when attending patients in their cottages, often without water or proper lighting. But I was astonished how seldom one saw a case of infection. Probably the risk of infection would have been greater if the mother had been moved to hospital and out of her own environment where she had acquired immunity to the germs in her own home. Mothers did not need to be encouraged by advice to breast feed their babies for it was cheaper and easier than the only alternative which in those days was cow's milk. From a medical point of view there were other reasons for encouraging breast feeding; one was the prevalence of tuberculosis and other diseases in cows, so their milk was therefore a danger to the health of young babies in particular, and the other reason was that pasteurisation had not yet arrived on the scene, and the only way to make the milk safe was by boiling. Even after boiling the facilities in the home for keeping milk and feeding bottles away from dust and flies were sadly lacking.

As soon as the baby was born it was bound round its middle with a roll of flannel and tightly wrapped in a shawl over a woollen nightdress, with only its mouth and nose showing; its little arms and legs were quite immobilised for the first few weeks. This method was also customary in other parts of the country. The baby spent the first week or even more without going out of doors, often in a wooden cradle that could be rocked. These old cradles have now disappeared but no doubt that 'rocking the baby' did no harm and often

induced sleep.   There were many cases of intestinal
disorders probably due to infected milk and poor
hygiene, but on the whole these country born infants
were healthier than those born and brought up in the
poorer parts of the big cities.

It was the usual practice at this time to keep a
mother in bed for nine or ten days following her
confinement whether she was in hospital or in her
own home. This had not always been possible among
the poor of the large cities, and it was difficult to
persuade mothers in the country districts, especially
if it was not her first baby, to stay in bed for this
'lying in' period. I think they really preferred to
have their babies at home even had there been hospital
beds available, for they liked to feel they could still
have some control over day to day affairs;   however
they were tempted to get back to their housework and
often got up after a couple of days, apparently with
little ill effect.   Maybe they were ahead of medical
teaching, for today this 'lying in' period has been
discontinued and, unless there is some complication,
mothers are encouraged to get up after two or three
days.

* * * * *

In a country practice in the 1920's transport and
communications were great problems.   Although we
as doctors had our motor cars it was difficult for
patients to get to our surgery, except on market days
and on other days when special transport was available. Even so there were set routes along which the
buses ran, and it was no easy matter to reach the
route from outlying areas at the right time. When
patient and doctor did meet there was then the question
of medicine and possible hospital treatment. They had
great faith in a bottle of medicine. When visiting, we
always made an effort to carry many emergency med-

icines with us and these helped to keep the patients going. We did our own dispensing at the surgery for all our private patients, and for those panel patients who lived further than one mile from a chemist. If the patient had to be taken to the hospital which was over twenty miles away, ambulances were provided by the voluntary organisation, St John's Ambulance, which did excellent work as far as their resources could stretch. If there was not an ambulance available we had to take the patients ourselves. As well as transport difficulties there was also the question of communication, for telephones were few and far between. It often meant a long cycle ride or even a ride on horseback. Conditions in the houses were not conducive to good diagnosis of the patient's complaint especially after dark. Electricity had not arrived in the remote areas and accommodation in the cottages was very limited. When surgery, even of a minor nature, was required it became a matter of working under difficulties. I remember an occasion when I was called urgently to a farm ten miles in the country. At the time my younger farming brother happened to be with me and I persuaded him to keep me company. It appeared that a young man had run into a stone wall on his motor cycle and although he had done considerable damage to the skin and tissues of his thigh over a large area, luckily there was no bone injury. In the circumstances I had no choice but to proceed to clean up the leg and stitch the wound. Of course it was dark and my brother being the only available help had to hold the oil lamp while I operated. There was no anaesthetic available. Whilst working on the job I noticed the light was flickering and after a harsh word to my assistant I looked up just in time to catch the lamp before it and its holder had reached the floor. One might classify that as a hazard of home surgery! The case made an uninterrupted recovery.

Such was the background to our country practice.

We had no difficulty in getting staff, but it was not quite so easy to find suitable ones. We started with a chauffeur-gardener and a maid and as the practice grew in our third year we employed another maid to help with the two children, and a clerk-dispenser. Our life had to fit in with the convenience of our patients with the result that on market days and Saturdays we could never go far from the surgery except to visit serious cases or emergencies. Sunday afternoons we usually spent in visiting outlying districts, to pay periodic calls on some of our elderly patients who were unable to make the journey to see us in the town.

Having spent some years on the resident staff of a London teaching hospital, I found the lack of an emergency laboratory service and of X-ray facilities lack of transport aggravated the problem. We seriously considered establishing these services ourselves, for we had the accommodation available and had we finally decided to stay in private practice no doubt this would have happened. On the other hand we realised that with this addition to the services it would mean more of one's time devoted to administrative and consultative work and less to the care of our patients who were our chief concern. We had an example of this to a small extent when we engaged an assistant with a view to partnership to look after a branch practice we had acquired at Abersoch. The practice grew but so did 'second opinions' making life busier than ever and giving us even less time for our private life.

An example of the difficulties without a laboratory service stands out clearly in my memory. I was called out in the evening to a case of tonsilitis in a boy of seven. When I examined his throat I at once became suspicious that it might be the dreaded diphtheria and as he had a younger brother the problem was even more serious. I discussed my views with the parents and told them that the nearest reliable laboratory willing to give an immediate service to help my diagnosis at that time of night was a hundred miles away. However, they had a fast private car and the father volunteered to take the throat swab and to wait for the result of the examination. I warned them that this would only give an indication of the infection and that a culture would take a few more days to be sure of the result. However, after returning with the evidence from the laboratory the father was adamant that the first step in the treatment should be given at once. At four o'clock in the morning I was called back and although there was no certainty that he was suffering from diphtheria I gave a preventive dose of serum. Two days later the result came back negative. All this trouble had been worthwhile for had the result been different and no precautions taken we, the parents and myself, should have taken the blame. Some years later — still before immunisation had appeared on the scene — I saw young children in Bristol dying from this terrible disease.

I must not leave this account of medical service without referring to home nursing, which was indeed of immense importance, for there was insufficient hospital accommodation and this was too far from home for many cases. Trained district nurses were few and we have already told of their fine work, but there were usually young women available who were intelligent although untrained, who could be called on to help. Many of these young women devoted many years to looking after sick and aged relatives in their homes and many of them we have met recently, elderly spinsters who had sacrificed many years of their lives in such a good cause. They would be living in penury today were it not for private charities, and more recently a little help from the State.

There were four other medical practices in Pwllheli

besides our own. Although we never formed a group practice amongst ourselves — and we realised too well that we were all too individualistic for such to be a success — we worked very happily each one in his own way. The doctors were all highly esteemed by the townsfolk and in the surrounding countryside. Two of them in particular deserve special mention. One was Dr O. Wynne Griffith who had qualified in 1878 at Guys Hospital, London, and was still in practice in 1925 after 47 years of very active life. He died in 1947 at the ripe old age of 97. He had rendered a service unequalled in my opinion, to a population

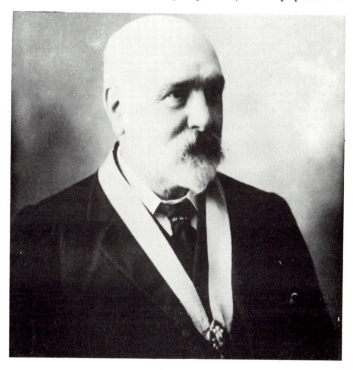

Doctor O. Wynne Griffith

scattered over 300 square miles.

In his earlier days, as I have already mentioned, he was known to be away from his surgery for days travelling around the country by horse and trap, visiting his patients. He always carried with him a dispensary of medicines and well equipped bags for any emergency. He is reputed to have travelled more than 800 miles a week many times. But that was not the only service he gave to the community. He was an elder of the Presbyterian Church for sixty years, Mayor of Pwllheli twelve times and received its honorary freedom for his services in 1932. He was also Chairman of the County School Council and an Alderman of the County Council. This must be a unique record hardly ever to be surpassed.

The other well known character was Dr Jones Evans who had qualified at Liverpool University in 1898 and died at the relatively young age of 68. He also had served the town well. He was an elder of the Church and a Justice of the Peace and had been Mayor of the town three times.

There is much truth in the old saying that if you want a job well and willingly performed look for a busy man.

Unqualified Practice

When we entered general practice there were two unqualified practitioners in our district. 'Unqualified Practice' is always looked upon by members of any profession with considerable discredit, not to say distaste. The qualified members having spent a number of years studying their subjects know full well that a newcomer who steps on the scene without such training must be misleading the public. Too often this attitude is mistaken by the general public as a fear of competition by the profession, as would be the case in the world of small business. Yet let us not forget that it was not until the middle of the 18th century — a little over two hundred years ago — that apprenticed surgeons were joining together to "foster a knowledge of the art of healing". It looks very close to me who by personal contact can reach back half way to that period.

We owe much in Wales in particular to bonesetters. Of course they made many mistakes for they were content to go only by rule of thumb as their predecessors had done for many centuries. As newer knowledge arrived from the research of great pioneers the weakness of the craft of the bonesetter became more apparent. Yet the famous Sir James Paget gave a lecture published in the British Medical Journal in 1867 on "Cases which bonesetters cure". Even the great Hugh Owen Thomas was descended from a family of bonesetters, but added much to their compendium of knowledge and skill by study and research. He

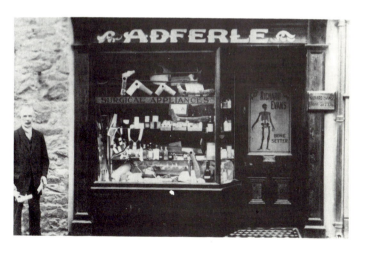

Pwllheli bonesetter

became a pioneer orthopaedic surgeon and was followed in his line by his nephew, Sir Robert Jones, one of the founders of modern bone surgery. Edward Jenner famous for his discovery of vaccination against smallpox, was only testing the veracity of the old folk tradition that an attack of cowpox protected against smallpox. So before condemning the remedy prescribed by an unqualified person, we should always examine the claim carefully and even test it, as long as the care of the patient takes first priority.

The two 'quacks' in our district were a bonesetter and a man who professed to cure 'wild warts'. I was never able to test the efficacy of their treatment. However, I had at the back of my mind the case of a relation, a young man who had an accident to his leg and who remained a cripple for the rest of his life. At the time of the accident he had been attended by a bonesetter. But in those days broken bones sometimes resulted in deformities even after treatment by qualified doctors, for there was no means of checking by X-rays to make sure the injury had been properly treated to effect complete repair. Sir Arthur Keith in his book "Menders of the Maimed" castigates members of his own profession for not keeping up to date, and concludes that as long as we have such members we deserve to have quacks.

We were very fortunate to be able to practice in such pleasant surroundings. It made our work more agreeable. Looking back I realise also that an even greater help was the fact that I had returned to practice in my native heath. The knowledge of the background of the families in his care is inestimable to the general practitioner. Careful study had shown, and it was an accepted fact, that heredity played an important part in longevity. I often heard country folk talk of the 'brittle' families, members of whom died before attaining old age or even when quite young. It is true that immunity to disease can be produced naturally or artificially but heredity also somehow plays its part. Much can be done by environment to enhance or suppress hereditary characteristics, but no environmental influences can change a racehorse into a shire horse or vice versa. I knew the family history of many of our patients and this fact helped us very much in our approach to their problems.

III. "UNDER THE CHERRY TREE" ONCE AGAIN

> Paid a golau'r lamp, mae'n gynnar;
>   Paid a thynnu'r lleni i lawr,
> 'Rwyf yn caru y cysgodion
>   A'u cyfaredd — dyma'r awr.
> > *Moelwyn*
> Do not light the lamp, it's early;
>   Let the fading daylight shine,
> For I am in love with shadows
>   And their spell — the hour is mine.
> > *Translated by Sir Thomas Parry Williams.*

Forty five years have passed by since our practice days in Pwllheli. We are now living at Cricieth on the outskirts of our practice area, and are free to explore the countryside and note the changes that have occurred in the meantime.

As we journeyed around the familiar places and visited old friends one picture had not changed. The mountains, hills and the sea still looked the same. Yr Eifl, with Tre'r Ceiri towering above my old home, Snowdonia with its rugged peaks and cascading waterfalls are as unperturbed as ever. As the great national poet, Ceiriog, noted a century ago, "the great mountains stand firm and the wind roars over them as loudly as ever."

It was only natural that in studying the changes that had taken place in the villages and lives of the people, I should return to the three villages associated with my childhood, and that have been described in the earlier part of this book.

Llanaelhaearn, except for a small, new housing estate in the village had altered very little at first sight. However there were many significant changes not at first apparent. The smithy had disappeared with its familiar sounds and picture of horses waiting patiently to be shod. The mill was no longer in use and the miller and his family have disappeared; the building had been converted into a modern dwelling house. With easier and quicker transport flour can now be purchased from further afield and the farmers either grind their own corn or sell it to merchants in the bigger towns. There is an excellent bakery in the village large enough to supply the local needs, and distribute its bread and cakes to a large area of the countryside. Services are still held in the Church but the old graveyard has a forlorn and neglected appearance. There is no resident Minister for the Chapel, but services are held regularly and a vestry room has been built for meetings connected with the Chapel. Sometimes the Vicar holds services in the Chapel and on occasions members of the Chapel attend services in the Church. The county authority has decided to close the school but the local inhabitants are protesting vigorously. The children would have to be taken by bus to Trefor should their school be forced to close.

With the improvement in the roads and transport facilities Llanaelhaearn appears much nearer to Caernarfon and Pwllheli, its market towns.

The population remains about the same but there are fewer children in a greater number of homes now that families are smaller. This is one reason given for the suggested closure of the village school.

Llannor has hardly changed at all except for a small estate of council houses and one or two new, privately owned bungalows. The village school closed many years ago and the children are now taken by bus to a larger school two miles away. The old post office is now derelict and its business has been transferred to a new house across the road.

Of the three villages, Efailnewydd has altered more than the other two. There are many new houses, both private and council owned, situated away from the main road. The old stone cottages still exist and many of them have been renovated and modernised. The tailor's workshop is now a dwelling house and the village Inn has no licence. The Chapel and its recently built Vestry are the focal point of village life and there is a resident Minister.

None of these villages has a playing field or any means of recreational activities either in or out of doors, with the exception of a village hall at Llanael-haearn. They all rely on Pwllheli for their amusements, be it sport, music or drama.

It is a pleasure when travelling today through many of the Welsh villages to see that the new houses and council estates have, on the whole, been well sited and the old ribbon development of former days when terraced houses, many without gardens, stretched the whole length of the village street has been avoided. There now seems to be far more pride in making the village an attractive place in which to live. The Women's Institute and Garden Clubs have done much to encourage this attitude. Recently the competition for the best kept village in Wales has also stimulated local effort. The small cabbage patch has been hidden by a colourful array of flowers and many flowering trees and shrubs have been planted. A South Caernarfonshire village has been successful in earning the title of the 'Best kept Village' several times in the last few years.

Some of the more isolated old stone cottages that I knew so well have disappeared, but others have been given a face-lift and extensions added, usually but not always in keeping with the old traditional style. Many

of these old homes have been rescued from dereliction
by English-speaking people as holiday homes or for
their retirement.   Some of these newcomers have
family links with Wales and take a great interest in
local affairs.   The acquisition of these old buildings
by strangers has not meant that the natives have been
driven away. The alternative would have meant leaving
cottages to become ruins.

But there are many changes in the countryside itself.
The Forestry Commission as well as local nurseries
and landowners have planted large and small forests
of the inevitable conifers. The lower slopes of Yr
Eifl are still bare of trees, but it is interesting to see
how the green fields and pasture land are spreading
up the hillside replacing the gorse, heather and
bracken. This change can be noticed in many parts of
the Llŷn Peninsula as the result of the successful
efforts of the hill farmers encouraged by government
help.   There are electricity pylons and power cables
crossing the land in many places, although the valley
below my old home has not yet been marred by their
unsightliness. I suppose the great benefits electric
power brings must outweigh their ugliness and we
must learn to live with them.

The old telegraph posts have disappeared in many
parts and the wires have been laid underground,
especially where places were exposed to gales and
snow. A favourite pastime for boys in my young days
was to press their ears to the posts to listen to the
sound like a distant roar and imagine the messages
sent from station to station.

The small fields with their hedges and stone walls
appear much the same as before. Apparently there
has been no hurry to enlarge the fields and scrub out
the hedges to make huge tracts of land as in Lincoln-
shire and other places in order to make cultivation
easier.   In all probability the narrow, windswept
valleys here need the protection of these walls and

hedges.

One of the most remarkable changes which I noticed was the absence of rabbits in fields that I remembered so well as being infested with this pest. Corn and hay crops had been devastated and the hedges and the banks torn up by burrows. Then nature sent a rabbit plague, myxomatosis, that cleared the countryside of these rodents and made the land productive once again. So many people are carried away by sentiment to the detriment of common sense, and fail to realise the fundamental truth that the struggle for existence is still going on. This struggle is not only between human beings but between all living matter — animals and plants. Those that are the fittest survive.

I remember once in Bristol receiving a letter from a person in Somerset, he also sent a copy to the press, pointing out my stupidity in fighting and campaigning to exterminate the common house fly. He said, quite rightly, that it was one of the best scavengers of dead animals and vegetation and so was a great help to nature itself. However, his information was not a balanced view for he did not point out its dirty habits so dangerous to living man and beast, or to the many diseases that it transplanted from one source to another.

I fear that there are signs of the return of the rabbit after the government had taken a hand in helping to check nature's way. I wonder if we realise that our methods of trapping, poisoning and shooting are not less cruel than their destruction by nature herself.

Of course road traffic has increased enormously, but all the roads are now tarmacadamed and many have been widened and dangerous corners straightened out. Even so the urge for speed by many drivers is frightening on our comparatively quiet country roads. My mind goes back to our practice days when on one occasion my wife was driving in the old bull-nosed Morris along the main Caernarfon road when a horse and trap ran into her from a side road. In those days it was expected that motorists should give way to animals and horsedrawn vehicles, but if they suddenly appeared from a side lane it was not always possible to take avoiding action. When the police sergeant interviewed Joan he asked what speed she was doing. "Oh," she said, "about twenty five miles an hour." "Please don't say that," he replied, "the legal speed limit is twenty miles an hour!" Fortunately there was no serious damage done to the car or the occupants of the trap.

The outward appearance of the stone farmhouses have not changed. Although the old hay barn, the stone built cowsheds and other buildings are still standing, they have been superseded by modern concrete and asbestos roofed buildings, more useful and hygienic but very different from the picture in my mind of the farmyard and its activities. Farming has

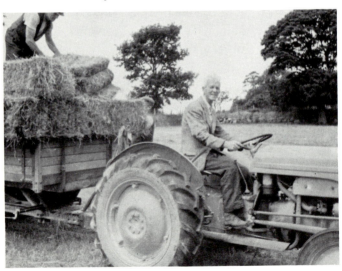

Tractor

certainly become a very different proposition from the occupation that I knew in my young days. I see great changes even since our practice days, for forty years have now passed by. No longer does one see the sower walking along the field sowing the grain or the labourer scything the hay. There are far more animals in the fields in spring and summer. In the old days the cattle were mostly Welsh blacks or short horns. Now one sees many Friesians and Herefords among the herds, and a larger breed of sheep, although the Welsh mountain sheep are even more numerous on the mountains. It is sad to see the disappearance of the heavy farm horses working the plough, and the horse drawn mower replaced by the tractor. The tractor and its attachments can do the work of many men using their old time tools. Now even the tractor has been replaced by the combine harvester on many farms to reap and thresh and leave the straw to be

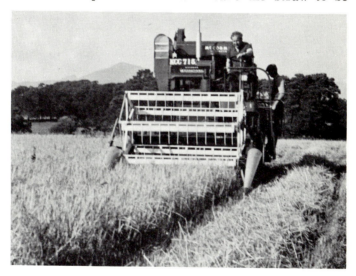

Combine harvester

dealt with by the mechanical binder or burnt. Drying methods have been introduced, and this counteracts the effect of rain at harvest time which used to mean so much additional work in the fields. It is only on the small farm that the farm labourer of old is still to be found. On most farms skilled mechanics are required to work the new machinery, and the different methods of handling livestock has resulted in specialisation by the staff. The winter care of animals in new or converted buildings which have been purpose-planned, helps to increase hygiene and save labour. All heavy work such as cleaning out the sheds is done mechanically, and the feeding of the stock has also been planned to reduce work to a minimum. This means that the stockman, the shepherd, and the engineer have to be trained in their special skills to replace the labourers of the past. Each plays his part in the team and accepts the responsibilities that devolve upon him in his day-to-day tasks. I gape and wonder what the grandfathers would have thought on many of these farms I have visited recently, if they could have seen the changes that have taken place during the last generation — the use made of electric power, the piped water and the many complicated machines. Is this all progress? Economically and under today's circumstances the answer must be yes. But with every change there is something missed. With bigger herds and more milking cows the days of Bess, Bet and Meg have gone, to be replaced by 'units'. One no longer hears two or three men discussing in the evening the merits or shortcomings of their charges. The stockman is a lone man and only summons help from an expert when something goes wrong. From time to time I get a feeling of warm nostalgia when I come across a smallholding that has not yet become 'up to date'!

But what a change this has meant to the farmer's wife. No longer is butter made at the farm, nor the

cows milked by hand.   The cows are milked with
electric machines, the milk is collected and taken in
tanks to the depot.   In fact the room that used to be
called the dairy is often now the home of a deep freeze
and of extra storage space for food. The wife now has
more time to spare from the old chores and I notice
that many have taken great interest in gardening and
improving the comforts of the home, as well as in
adding to the charm of its surroundings.

Many of the fundamental maxims which we accepted
in early life and on which we hoped to build have been
shattered by new thoughts, new discoveries and
scientific developments.   Many of these appeared to
be impossible in former days.   Such a thought must
have prompted the former Prime Minister of Israel,
Ben Gurion, to say that, "The person who believes in
miracles is a realist."

Unbelievable changes have taken place in the home
during the last fifty years, and the old folk who had
worked hard to bring up a family at the beginning of
the century would be at a loss to realise how much
could be accomplished by the turn of a switch! Gone
are the days of the kitchen range and its ovens, for
dealing with all the cooking and heating the water.
These had to be black-leaded and the flues frequently
cleared, taking up much time and toil to say nothing
of the dirt and dust that resulted. Washing day meant
many hours of hard labour — water to be heated in a
copper in the scullery or an outhouse, a mangle for
squeezing out the water, the scrubbing board and the
heavy irons that had to be heated on the fire. Not only
does the modern washing machine make life easier
for the housewife of today, but since the advent of
man-made fibres the clothing is so much easier to
launder. No longer are the children dressed in cotton
dresses, pinafores and frilled underwear that require
ironing, and the goffering iron for frills has now

become a 'museum piece'. In many of the working class homes the wife and mother now finds time to supplement the family budget by taking part-time jobs. There were compensations, however in the old days for the lack of modern facilities because labour was cheap and readily available for the middle class family. Often a washerwoman would be employed for one day a week to cope with the family washing and ironing. The day-to-day tasks of looking after the children and running the home could be shared by helpers either resident or daily.

Perhaps one of the greatest changes that a housewife of one or two generations ago would notice would be the change in shopping and the packaging of food. One still finds the village shop in the small hamlets sufficient for the daily necessities but even these now have a supply of frozen foods and dried vegetables, so that there is less reliance on daily supplies of fresh food, and a greater variety of goods on display. In the towns I think our Edwardian forbears would miss the personal attention of the small shopkeeper, who is gradually being ousted by the self-service supermarkets with their rows and rows of tinned foods, plastic containers and packeted goods of all kinds — all very handy and time-saving no doubt, but there is no time or opportunity for a chat while the grocer weighs out half a pound of butter, sugar, oatmeal and the rest.

There are, of course, advantages and disadvantages in the pre-packing of food and other household articles. Factory packing in these days of high labour costs should make distribution cheaper and less wasteful, but there is need for a thorough investigation to be made into the cost of packaging because it must influence the price of the actual product. It is also very necessary to have packages properly labelled regarding quality and quantity so that the housewife is not misled. That applies also to toilet articles and medical supplies. Much has been done by the

Consumer's Council and others but more can still be
done to safeguard the shopper.

'Plastics' and Their Uses

Joan and I have been indirectly interested in the
scientific development of plastics because her father
made a notable contribution through his chemical
researches over fifty years ago.   Like many other
scientific research workers he did not become
involved in their commercial exploitation, although
he had great confidence in their future possibilities.
If he had survived to see how much they are used
today even he would have been amazed to see the
many and varied ways in which plastics are now used.
They now play an enormous part in changing the
habits of the people, and even the mode of life in
every home in the country.

From the farmers' angle they have helped to make
work on the farm very much easier. Fertilisers and
feeding stuffs now arrive in plastic bags which protect
the contents from the weather and vermin.   These
bags need not be stored under cover and therefore do
not occupy valuable space in farm buildings. Polythene
piping has made it possible to carry water to distant
fields without the help of skilled engineers or plumbers,
for it is easy to handle, and no deep trenches have to
be made, for frost will not damage the pipes as
happened with the old iron ones. The work can now
be carried out by the farmer himself, or one of his
workers who is usually capable of doing the job. No
longer need the hayricks be covered by tarpaulins or
thatched. A few sheets of polythene, usually black
and well tied down give adequate protection against
the weather for a long while and do not deteriorate
like sacking. Valuable heavy equipment is often
protected by covering with this completely waterproof
material, and it can be used as a protection for

animals when there is a shortage of farm buildings.
A temporary shelter can be made as a lambing pen
during inclement weather. The horticulturist is
making more and more use of plastics to replace
glass in greenhouses, and for frames and cloches
which are much easier to handle, with a considerable
saving in breakages. Plastic pots are gradually
replacing the old clay pots for they are lighter to use,
easier to clean and breakages are far fewer. As well
as helping the farmers and market gardeners, the
builder often finds use for plastic sheeting in many
ways, especially to protect a site from the weather so
that routine work can continue. There seems to be no
branch of industry where plastics have not penetrated
to replace glass or metal. At the present time there
is one great disadvantage to plastic containers. Their
two merits, imperviousness to water and resistance
to decay, means that their disposal creates difficulty
and they can become a nuisance. In its lighter form
it can be easily burnt but the heavier containers such
as bottles, cans and bags, resist heat and we find
them in abundance on our beaches, discarded by
picnickers or thrown from ships. The hedgerows and
fields are also dumping grounds for this unwanted
rubbish, and this type of litter is not only a health
menace to man and beast, but owing to the gaudy
colours used by the manufacturers, it is an unnecessary
eyesore.

Pollution of the Environment

In recent years it has given me much pleasure to see
the new outlook of government towards pollution of
the environment.

I had spent a good part of my life in the battle-front
facing this problem, and often found myself up against
the stone wall of central governments. I remember
more than one attempt being made in Bristol to

prevent pollution and they were stifled in the 'national interest'. Officialdom repeated parrot-like a northern adage, "Where there's muck there's money." We know too well that such thoughts arose from ignorance. When studying the problem of slum clearing I realised that those dwellings had been erected in congested masses so that people should be "near their work." We, the Public Health staff, had the job of condemning them and pulling them down to allow a little fresh air and cleanliness into the neighbourhood. Today almost the same arguments are produced for locating industry near dwellings both in town and country, whereas this should be tackled as the task of transport.

In all this matter of guarding the environment the question of water may be the first priority. I realised the importance of this on visits to the Middle East and indeed in other parts of the world. We realised to the full its importance in this country during the war, when the water supply of some centres of population were bombed. I need not here refer to all the uses we make of water to keep us healthy — in the homes, in public baths, for conveniences, on farms and for horticulture to mention but a few. Conservation of water is an essential part of planning to supply an adequate flow of clean water to the homes and for industry.

Disposal of sewage is very important. It is incredible that in 1972 it is still necessary to bring home to local authorities the fact that sewage should be rendered harmless before its disposal into rivers or the sea. I wonder if it is realised how many seaside towns, villages and houses are still turning crude sewage into the sea. In former days when I used to raise this matter I was told that the advisers of the Ministry of Health were satisfied that if there was a certain dilution of the sewage there was no risk to bathers! My blunt reply was that bathing in sewage, however diluted, was never aesthetic or healthy. The

time must come soon to compel treatment of all crude
sewage before it is dispersed into rivers or the sea.
When I was a young Medical Officer of Health the
friendly Town Clerk, Josiah Green, often reminded
me of the 70,000 unflushed toilets in the City of
Bristol. My retort was always the same — that it
was no worse than turning the crude sewage into the
river Avon. For several consecutive years I went
with a survey boat to test the pollution of that river,
and invariably we found that there was so much
pollution that there was not enough oxygen to give fish
a chance of survival within two miles of the port of
Avonmouth. In addition there was also industrial
pollution. This happened on a tidal river with a rise
and fall of nearly thirty feet which ought to have
driven the poisonous waste materials out to sea.
Some years ago the Bristol City Council bravely
tackled the problem, and I have reason to believe that
before long there will be fishing in the Avon once again.

Twenty years ago at a conference on smoke pollution
I noted with regret that the Bristol authority had
decided to scrap the electric trams and replace them
with diesel buses. Recently I was interested to see
on television that the New Vienna has been planned to
bring back the electric trams as public transport in
order to reduce atmospheric pollution.

Although the atmospheric pollution in our big towns
has vastly improved, we must watch that factories are
not built near the peoples' homes; transport to work
is no longer a problem. The misinformed do not
realise that there can be more danger from poisonous
vapours driven out by fans than from dust and smoke
from high chimneys. Nor is it always remembered
that stagnant moist air, such as occurs at some
seaside towns accentuates the danger.

There is one feature of very great importance to
our crowded little island. It is our beaches and sea
coast. More than ever our children and grandchildren

will be depending on their beaches as recreational 'parks'. It is not enough to state that the beaches are free up to high water mark when access through many sand dunes has been closed as private property. In some places car parks have invaded the beach, and the danger to bathers from speed boats has already meant bathing fatalities, to say nothing of the fumes from their engines. All these threats to our beaches must be controlled before it is too late, and it might be wise to insist that all land for at least two hundred yards from high water mark should be made public property and left free from building in the future.

We are fortunate in living in an environment relatively free from pollution, but even so there are warning signs that the problems facing the big cities may invade the countryside unless steps are quickly taken to curb the modern 'spoilers'. There are legacies from the past, and some more recent, that have left their scars. The slag heaps and derelict slate quarries are but examples. Attempts are being made here and there to cover up the eyesores and encourage vegetation to return. Our beaches are being spoilt by oil washed up by the sea, and insoluble debris like plastic containers and other material. There is a hopeful sign that the younger generation is becoming aware of this menace for I heard recently that the Girl Guides have volunteered to clear the beaches, in our part of the coast at least, regularly during the summer months.

No one is anxious to see more and more legislation, so let us hope that voluntary effort on the part of all concerned and common sense public opinion will prevail before governments have to intervene.

Education in the Village School

Education is very much a subject for discussion and in people's thoughts today. It was always of great importance in Welsh homes, and I have already mentioned the difficulties, mostly economic, that stood in the way of further education to children from ordinary families. This matter of finance was always uppermost in the parents' minds when they strove to give their children a better start in life than they had had. In these same rural areas money is no longer a problem, for the state provides the requirements in the form of facilities and grants. At the present moment the villagers are very concerned about the closure of village schools. The teachers in these schools, men or women, who for the most part were highly successful in their work, not only had the

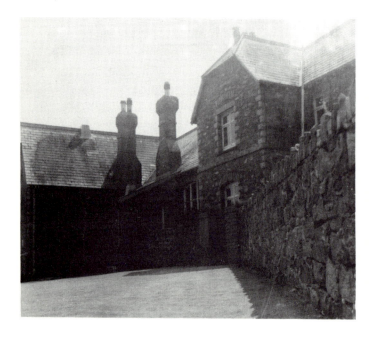

Village school, Llanhaelhaearn

confidence of the children, but took an active part in the life of the village. The older folk in the village feel that an important, and to some of them, a vital part of village life is removed when the school is closed. The children will be away from the village for the whole day if they have to go further afield to another school.

From the point of view of the authorities on the other hand there are many advantages in establishing a bigger school to provide for the needs of several villages to replace the individual ones the children have been attending. The size of families in rural areas has diminished rapidly in recent years so there are fewer children attending these small schools. The expense of keeping them for a few children has increased enormously, with increased salaries to the staff, heating and maintaining the building, and the provision of reserve staff in case of sickness or for special occasions. Added to this is the risk of having an unsuitable head for a small school without an alternative, for it is not easy to correct such a mistake in public life. Today the problem of transport for the children, although adding to the cost, is relatively unimportant with a bus to take the children from a scattered area, whereas in the past it would have been impossible for the children to make such daily journeys. There is a sharp division of opinion between the Education Authority and the villagers over the closing of these schools. One cannot, however, agree that if the decision goes against the villagers it is undemocratic to override their views if they have had an opportunity to express them. The Authority is responsible by law to provide an education service with money provided from the public, and not from the villagers only. However it is sad to see, as we travel through the smaller hamlets and villages these schools shut and not put to any other use. It certainly does contribute to the moribund appearance of these places especially during daytime.

The comprehensive school is far from being wholly accepted. I have already referred to the disease of 'bigness' and this has certainly affected education administrators. There must be a decision made regarding the optimum size of any school. From the sentimental angle the merging of schools which have had a high reputation for centuries brings much sadness, and the result of the change is often to be regretted.

Nothing could be further from the truth than the idea that all men are born equal, and yet it is becoming the basis of all ideas on education and society today. I believe that every child will develop according to his innate ability together with the assistance he receives from outside. The authorities today argue that the progress of the child depends on how the child is taught and on his environment. Do they ignore the fact of his or her innate ability? Do they believe that the arguments put forward in the breeding of animals can apply to human beings? A point that is often forgotten by the sentimentalist in his enthusiasm for the under-privileged, whether by God or man, is the fact that the future of our country depends on the quality of its citizens. The education system certainly must not forget the talented young people, for they are possible leaders of the future. There is much more knowledge available today than in my school days, and there are improved methods of imparting it. Nevertheless, there are many complaints that the teaching of the basic three R's is being neglected because of experimentation and extra demands upon the teacher.

I have been interested in education all my life, not only as a student but as a parent, teacher, and as a School Medical Officer for thirty years.

In 1959 I visited Iran as a consultant for the World Health Organisation to report on the teaching of

Preventive Medicine in that country and to make suggestions regarding its future administration. There were certain lessons to be learned from my study of the organisation I found in that country. The Iranian Government placed education in the front line of the national policy. They considered the problem so urgent that they had not waited to train the necessary staff or build the accommodation necessary to meet the consequent expansion. In the ordinary schools in many areas in Teheran they had arranged a shift system for the pupils and many classes were held in the open air, in the school grounds. I was particularly interested in the University training of medical students. The Shah had decided, so I was told, on advice from his counsellors that the number of medical students must be trebled, as there were not enough doctors in Iran. In Teheran they had therefore an annual intake of three hundred students at the medical school. The largest lecture theatre could only hold one hundred, so all lectures had to be duplicated and it was a case of first come, first served! The Persian student is very intelligent and has a good memory, so that with the aid of good notes very few failed to qualify. I was unable to find out what happened to the clinical teaching, but they certainly did not attach the same importance to that aspect of medical training as we do in this country. But what happened to these young doctors after they had qualified? The villages I saw were very inadequately supplied with doctors, nurses or health inspectors. The result was that many of these doctors, with the help of scholarships or by other means found their way to other countries and many never returned. As I bluntly stated to the Chief of the medical school, "There are cheaper ways of exporting your best brains than by training them as doctors."

In my report to the World Health Organisation I recommended a central body (a Higher Institute) for the whole country, limited in its responsibility to dealing with all branches of Public Health. The duties of that body should be to choose a syllabus according to the need of the country, and review the requirements from year to year. It should also keep a register of all qualified persons and, most important of all, make itself responsible for finding jobs for them all. I understand that in the last twelve years many improvements on these lines have been made in Iran.

Could not such a scheme be applied to this country? Why should not the universities train to meet the demands from all branches of industry and the professions? It would be much better than training too many for one career leading to the surplus being unemployed, or too few to meet the requirements of another trade or profession. We have been troubled in the past by the 'brain drain' and I wonder how much is still taking place? We could do well to tackle this problem with advantage to the whole country, including our own rural community.

It can be argued that education has other purposes than that of training for an occupation. However in this material and highly competitive age we must acknowledge that the chief purpose of education is to train a young person to earn a living. Finding a suitable job to satisfy his own requirements and that of his family, is without doubt most important.

There should be a place for discipline in education and this includes self-discipline. The few loud protestations come from a small minority and are not always laudable in their purpose. The protestors should not be ignored lest they become dangerous to the liberty of those, and they are many, who act and think rationally.

The Influence of Religion

During the last two or three decades there seems to

have been an apparent decline in religion. Maybe, however, it would be truer to say that the decline is in the influence of religious establishments rather than in the belief and practice of Christ's teaching. In my youth the commanding influence of the Church and Chapel was the most important factor in the social life of the village. We all conformed to the code of conduct as set by these establishments. Those who conformed most readily were the Non-Conformists.

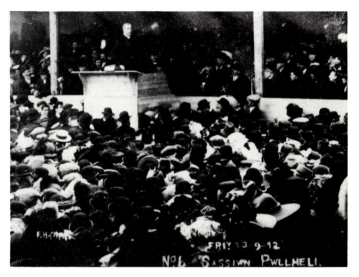

Open air preaching meeting in 1912

Of course there was a good deal of hypocrisy, but the vast majority were sincere believers in Christianity as they had been taught by their Ministers. It set the pattern of social behaviour and offered reward or punishment in after life according to one's deserts. Few people appeared to us as children to doubt this theory, and we were brought up within this code. Breaking the strict laws of behaviour as set forth by the religious bodies brought a reaction from the local

community that few could face. I am, of course, only
describing my impression of a small rural community.
The standards set in big towns and cities were very
different and varied considerably.

Today it is difficult to estimate the influence of
Church and Chapel on these rural villages. Certainly
during the last seventy years many factors have played
their part in disturbing the placid life of country folk.
The access to more money thereby raising the
standard of living is probably one reason, for it has
given more independence of thought and action.
Increased knowledge, too, in all branches of learning
has filtered through to the man in the street. Even
greater influence in this decline has been the teaching
of science to the children in school and the young
people at the universities. Radio and television have
reached most homes and have tremendous influence
on young and old — not always for the best.

How do the average parents today look at the religion
which they have adopted without question for most of
their lives? A few days ago the mother of two
daughters, one married and one working away from
home said with sadness that both had 'opted out'.
Could it be that later they will return to the fold?
Will the influence of 'the roots' and training at home
be sufficiently powerful to smother the newer ideas
about living? I have watched in our garden lovely
plants with variegated leaves suddenly producing a
strong branch of green leaves. If this latter growth
is allowed to continue the attractive variegated foliage
will gradually disappear, ousted instinctively by the
old root stock.

I am reminded of a story I heard about a doctor
colleague who was giving an address at the graveside,
at the funeral of his patient who had been ill for a long
time. The doctor was carried away by his own
eloquence (the 'hwyl' as it is called in Welsh) and he
spoke of the departure of the old man to the land

flowing with milk and honey, where there is no more pain, suffering or poverty, where there is sunshine and song for all eternity. One young man listening turned to his friend standing near and said, "I can't understand the doctor talking like that; why then did he try his best to keep him away from all these pleasures and let him suffer for so long?" No, we cannot influence the thinking of young people today as in the days of my youth by sentimental poetry deprived of sound reasoning and scientific truths.

I understand that communists describe all religions as opiates that help to deprive people of initiative towards progress.

Most people in this country disagree with this rash and wild statement. In public life during fifty years I was in close touch with all classes of people with different backgrounds and different religions. I watched many enthusiastic Christians who were not satisfied with voluble academic discussions of schemes which resulted in no action. Their thoughts and deeds did much to make their little world a happier place.

A verse by Robert Burns comes to my mind:

"When ranting round in pleasure's ground
Religion may be blinded;
Or if she gives a random sting
It may be little minded;
But when on life we're tempest driven,
A conscience but a canker —
A correspondence fix'd wi' heaven
Is sure a noble anchor."

The Cult of 'Bigness'

Before leaving Bristol I had been engaged in the changes associated with the new National Health Service. The need for considerable extension of the hospital services, and for more doctors to be trained became of paramount importance. But gradually I came to realise that those in authority were convinced that nothing was efficient unless it was big. Big hospitals of a thousand or more beds could afford more equipment and more specialists in a greater number of departments. In the Medical school of the University the class of students whom I taught as Professor of Public Health jumped in size from under twenty to over forty, and more staff were necessary for teaching. The fact that was overlooked was that overheads grew with the greater size, more supervisors were required and many of the best clinical specialists found themselves involved for a considerable part of their time, in committee and administrative work, thus depriving the patients of the services of the most valuable experts. When my University class grew to forty or more, I soon realised that I had no chance of getting to know them individually. They all became members of the class. Yet when I was a medical student the part I appreciated most at the Middlesex Hospital, was when my specialist chief took personal interest in me, which he could do when there was only a few in his class at the bedside. For the individual student these changes appeared to be retrograde, but I put the blame on the extension of the medical services following the Health Act to provide a National Medical service. When, however, we retired to our little farm I realised that the disease of 'bigness' had invaded farming. When I was a child Mr Lloyd George had made an historic speech on the subject of our debt to small nations. He also had stressed the importance of the smallholdings to keep the young people from deserting the countryside and escaping to the towns. Even recently reports have been published to show that production per acre was much higher in small units than on the big industrial farms. Today the language is very different. Economic factors, viability, complicated and expensive machinery are the primary considerations.

In the earlier part of the book I have referred to the

value of the smallholding to the part-time worker, enabling him to bring up a healthy family interested in the running of a home with a few acres to manage. How can one evaluate that aspect of husbandry? If there ever was a Royal Commission needed, here is a suitable subject for investigation — how to get the maximum production and utilise our limited land resources in an island that is rapidly becoming over-populated.   This investigation would have to take into consideration the health and contented living conditions of the people.   There must be an optimum size for every organisation, if it could only be found.   This problem of 'bigness' arises not only in education, health, industry and farming but also seems to be affecting art, music, architecture and even sport.

The modern artists no longer think in terms of producing pictures to hang in the home.   Rather do they feel the need to 'express themselves' on vast canvasses or murals, often controversial, for public display.   This also applies to sculpture, for one sees huge blocks of stone conceived and created in various forms, meaningless to many people both young and old, but who are persuaded to value them because the artists are trying to break away from old traditions. The French Impressionist generation of artists did make a break from the style of their predecessors, but they were not appreciated in their lifetime. Today the painter or sculptor with new ideas and efficient publicity finds that his or her work brings substantial financial rewards during his or her lifetime.   One wonders if their work will be appreciated and increase in value in years to come, as in the case of the old masters.

Modern music to be successful has to attract thousands of young people to 'Pop Festivals' or sell thousands of records.   The music makers become rich, for the young generation of today has more money to spend, and can afford to indulge themselves in rapid changes in fashion as well as in music. In the past the young folk tended to follow the fashion and ideas of their elders, but now they are more independent in all ways and can lead rather than follow.

Sport, especially football, attracts enormous crowds and vast stadiums have had to be built to accommodate the spectators. The need for more opportunities for young people to take part rather than be onlookers in athletics, swimming and other sports is appreciated, but necessary facilities are sadly lacking in many parts of the country, both in the rural and urban areas. However, there are hopeful signs that these shortcomings are gradually being met.

Modern Communication

In the earlier part of the book I have told of the almost self-sufficiency of the little village community in its day-to-day existence. There were certain essentials which had to be obtained from outside and in order to pay for these there had to be 'exports' from the community. But the cobbler, the grocer, the black-smith and the carpenter and others provided the requirements of the villagers. If these craftsmen and shopkeepers were to obtain their necessary materials then means of communication with the outside world was essential, and the roads provided these. Walking, or on horseback, had been the usual way to travel, the horse and cart and the bicycle then came along to hasten the journeys, and then the trains and buses revolutionised communications. When the Romans invaded Britain they were clever enough to realise that an easy and quick means of reaching these communities was necessary, not only for military purposes but to break down their independence. In later years, as roads and transport have improved, so villages have joined in looking for a central supply depot — the market town — and the villages have become less self-contained.

In the last twenty years, the transport system has changed immeasurably and has had a remarkable effect on family life. The enormous increase in the number of cars has demanded better and straighter roads, shortening the distances between different parts of the country. But like all progress this has led to certain drawbacks. Public transport including trains and buses have become less popular and are not always economically self-supporting. But they do provide an essential service for those who cannot use or afford a private car. Herein, therefore, lies another problem for the immediate future, as the roads and streets of our towns are gradually becoming incapable of satisfying the demand of the growing number of private cars. As I see it, there is but one solution to this problem, and it is the return of public transport to its proper status in the communication system.

Today with modern methods of air travel and the telephone, the world seems to have become smaller. When I was a young lad the departure of friends and relations who had decided to emigrate to America or Australia often meant that they would never return to the old country. Letters took many weeks to reach them and journeys by sea were long and often hazardous. Now these journeys can be taken in a few hours by plane, and the long distance telephone system enables parents to talk to their children in distant lands. More than any other new development the telephone has shortened the distance, and helped to keep families in touch with each other both in this country and abroad. A few months ago I answered the 'phone and was surprised to hear the voice of an American friend from whom I had not heard for some time. Thinking he might be visiting this country I asked him where he was speaking from and had the astonishing reply that he was 'phoning from his ranch in California! His voice sounded clearer than one often hears on local calls.

A Persian friend I met recently who was spending some weeks in London told me that he spoke to his mother in Teheran once a week. Forty five years ago when telephones were few, we installed a speaking tube from our front door to the bedside, so that anyone arriving on foot or on bicycle could rouse us in an emergency. I am reminded of a story told me by another doctor whose wife answered a call on the speaking tube from bed soon after he had settled down to sleep after a very tiring day. He whispered to her, "Say that I am out," and when she repeated the message the voice from the other end of the tube answered, "Well, the man you are sleeping with will do." To save his wife's reputation he had to respond to the call! Today for business purposes and in private homes the telephone is regarded as a necessity, and even the poorer housing districts are supplied with telephone kiosks. The use of the telegram as a quick means of communication as far as the general public is concerned, is almost a thing of the past, and one seldom sees the telegraph boy on his bicycle.

I was in the Royal Air Force when Alcock and Brown flew the Atlantic in 1919. Since those far off days, flying has become the usual method of reaching distant lands. Shipping is now almost entirely used for carrying cargoes or for pleasure cruises, and the person who needs to travel to distant lands to visit relations or for business purposes, finds air travel a saving both in time and money. There are drawbacks, and I think important ones, in the sudden change in temperature as one travels from north to south and the time factor in travelling from east to west. The human body has difficulty in adapting to these rapid changes as I and my daughter have both experienced.

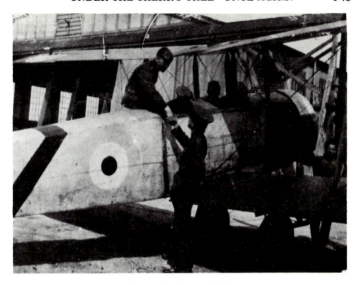

Royal Air Force, 1919

I left Athens on a hot, sunny day in late spring and was in Bristol in my office later that same day. I had to have a fire and found it took me a few days to acclimatise to the change. My daughter Eira had similar experiences when she was working in Nigeria, and flew home so as to have more time at home, although she always felt the need afterwards for a few days' rest in which to recover. The routine of the body is equally upset by the change in rhythm of eating and sleeping when travelling from east to west, and as air transport is becoming more and more rapid these factors will deserve more consideration. Long distance air travel is better organised than travelling from place to place in this country unless one has one's own car. It took me longer to travel from Prestwick in Scotland to Bristol than it did to cross the Atlantic from Montreal. It should be possible to alter this state of affairs, or may it possibly be the case that 'the shoemaker's shoes are in the greatest need of repair'?

The rapid spread of information has undoubted disadvantages. We become aware of crises of national, international and even personal family ones far too soon. In many cases these crises had solved themselves in the past before they had come to our knowledge, and so saved us unnecessary concern or worry. In truth people may one day see the wisdom of 'turning a deaf ear' to so much talk on the communication media.

Mr Lyons, the Prime Minister of Australia told me how his predecessor, William Hughes who was very deaf and used a hearing aid was sometimes seen to remove this aid deliberately when someone in Parliament, in committee or in a conference was making a long or dreary speech. It usually had the desired effect!

A few years ago some bright person or persons came up with the idea of a 'generation gap' as an explanation of the disturbed social attitude of a small minority of the younger folk. He thought that from this conception would come the understanding of the problem and the overcoming of the difficulties that had arisen. In fact there are, and always have been age groups, each with their own problems when they are facing life in all its aspects. Each group merges with time and living into the next group, but surely there can be no gap. The wise man in the Bible said that there is nothing new under the sun. The babies' tasks in growing up are concerned with learning to walk and talk and are very different from those of the school children. So it is through all the stages of man to old age. Medical practitioners are very much aware of this when they deal with the problem of immunisation against disease. No sooner have they completed their task with one group than time has delivered into their hands another lot of new arrivals which have to be dealt with in the same way.

Old Omar Khayam had his own ideas. This picture taken of a Persian miniature with the original words written in Persian around the margin illustrates his views.

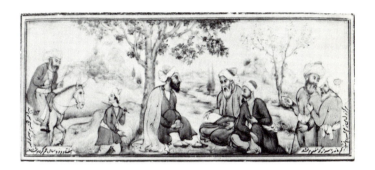

Persian miniature (Omar Khayam)

The young man sets out on his way through life: during the journey he meets wise men and discusses with them the way of life and living: then when old age arrives he realises how little he really knows.

Growth of wisdom and knowledge is a gradual process; that applies as equally to a free community as it does to the free individual.

A few years ago a Christmas message came from a friend, Doctor George Darling, Chief of the American Atomic Bomb Commission in Hiroshima. The greeting in the letter made a happy impression on my mind. It started with the words, "Today is the first day of the rest of your life...." How true this is! We can start

each day anew with more experience from the past.
We can follow the same path fortified by this experience
or we may change our direction. We may even decide
to slacken our pace and find time to stand and stare.

Modern Farming

In the last few years I have been able to visit many of
the old farms I knew from the days of my youth. I
found that farming in this part of the world was still
a way of life, and not the factory or business undertaking that seems to be revolutionising the industry
in other parts of the land. The farms are still about
the same size, 100 to 200 acres, either with owner
occupiers or tenant farmers, many in the hands of
the same families I had known. But there were great
changes in the methods of husbandry.

Sixty years ago in 1912, I spent a memorable
holiday on a farm on the side of Mynydd Cennin which
faced south west with a fine panoramic view of the
countryside stretching down to Cardigan Bay almost
ten miles away. I was sixteen years old and had just
matriculated and was soon to become a medical
student at the University. My health had not been too
good and my mother felt that three months spent on a
hill farm with plenty of good food was just what I
needed.

Until I returned I had lost touch with the family,
but about ten years ago I visited this farm and found
that my old friend, the son of the farm and my holiday
companion was now the present owner. He was in his
late sixties and very much of a cripple. When he was
a young man he had smashed his lower right leg
between a cart and the stone gatepost when trying to
stop a runaway horse. The local bonesetter had been
called in; he was left with a deformed foot and ankle
and had suffered much pain as a result ever since.
He told me that when his parents died the family had

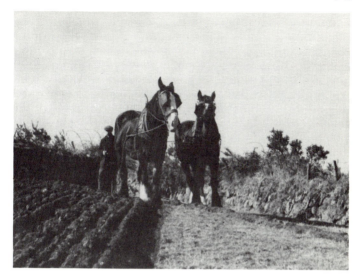

Horse ploughing

split up, the younger son had found another farm and his sister had married and left home. He had been left alone, with a housekeeper and two men to help on the farm. The family capital had been divided up so there was little left for him except the farm and a little stock. Those days before the war had not been easy ones for farmers. He married late in life and his only son, Geraint, was born in 1942 when he was fifty seven.

We talked about the old days and he brought back memories of life in the home and on the farm so long ago. It was a small hill farm of 130 acres, thirty acres of boggy and wet land down in the valley, thirty acres only fit for grazing sheep on the mountainside, and the remaining seventy acres that it was possible to cultivate to varying degrees. His father and mother were over sixty years old when I had been staying with them, and they and their three children (two boys and a girl) all worked on the farm with additional help at harvest time. That year the weather had been very warm and sunny throughout the summer and I too was able to enjoy the harvesting. Electricity and petrol had not arrived so the power needed was supplied by man, horse and dog! They had at least four horses, making two teams for the ploughing and harvesting. It was very hard and slow work with the horse and cart on the sloping land. In this respect it was very much like my old home at Uwchlawrffynnon. They had twelve milking cows and sixteen heifers reserved for the dairy herd. In addition they bred bullocks which were sold as stores when they were two and a half to three years old. In all they had about fifty five head of cattle. They also had a flock of eighty Welsh mountain ewes. The farm work had been laborious. The whole output of milk was churned to make butter and sold to the local shops. There had been no water-

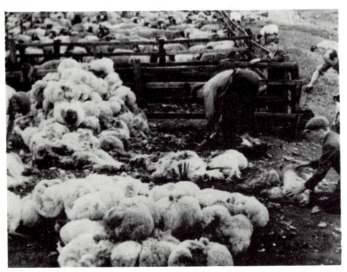

Shearing in 1912

wheel, not even horse power, and the small churn had to be turned by hand, and almost every day was butter-making day.

There was a hay barn where the hay could be carted and kept under cover, but two corn ricks had to be prepared so that one could be threshed immediately after the harvest and the other, threshed later in the autumn, had to be thatched for protection against the weather. The nearest railway station was five miles away and all the goods they needed such as coal, lime or basic slag had to be carted from the station. In order to save coal they used to cut peat from their own land, and I remember that the old fireplace in the kitchen was specially built for its use. Winter time had meant very hard work for all the family and preparations had to be made beforehand. Swedes, mangolds and potatoes had to be stacked ready for the animals and in addition hay, straw and gorse had to be chaffed for their food. There was also the job of getting rushes and straw for their bedding, cutting the rushes and harvesting them for this purpose. All the animals as well as the family had depended mostly upon food produced on the farm. There was plenty of running water in the fields, but for the house and farm buildings they had to draw their water daily from a pump near the house.

Recently I visited the farm once again. I found Geraint is now the present owner, and I am grateful to him for telling me what has been happening since I was last there, and the changes he had been able to make. Whilst he was still at school he had to bear the brunt of the work on the farm with the help of one man and his mother because his father had been a cripple for so long. Eight years ago, when he was twenty one, his father died and he found himself in complete charge of 100 acres, for thirty acres of the wet land in the valley had been bought by the Forestry Commission, drained and planted with trees. Most of the changes he showed me had been accomplished by him single-handed. Once or twice in the intervening years he had thought seriously of selling up for, as he said, there is much in favour of a weekly wage packet with no worries or problems when life is so short. As time passed, however, this attitude became gradually displaced by one of pleasure in his achievements, and he was now almost satisfied that his present life was really worth while.

Electricity had arrived at the farm twenty years ago, and had made a world of difference to the comfort of the home and to the work on the farm, especially on dark winter nights by giving light for the farm buildings. Gradually during the years the house had been equipped with an electric cooker, washing machine, refrigerator, a vacuum cleaner and television as well as electric fires. However, they are so exposed to the weather that it is essential to have an alternative method of heating and lighting in the form of a paraffin cooker, candles and lamps, and they still have a small coal fire. The telephone now brings them into touch with their friends, suppliers and customers, and saves them much time and travel.

He has no horses or carts; they have been displaced by the tractor, and its attachments have also replaced the old farm equipment. Even for cleaning out the buildings he uses mechanical means, and so too for carrying and handling the manure. The dairy herd is no more, indeed no milking is done, and they have to buy butter. They miss this especially as he now has been married for five years and has two children, a boy and a girl.

He does very little ploughing or cultivating of the land except for occasional reseeding. In the last two years however, he has given over five acres every year for growing swedes to feed the animals in the autumn. It would have been an eye-opener to his father, as it was to me, to see how easily this was done. The five acres were ploughed and cultivated in the spring and manured with a complete fertiliser as necessary. Three weeks were allowed to pass for all the weeds to germinate and then the field was sprayed with paraquat. The swede seeds were then sown as soon as possible with a precision drill. The crop was not weeded at all nor was it lifted when ripe, but instead the animals were turned on to the field to eat their ration, limited only by an electric fence. By such means Geraint reckoned to add about a hundred tons of good maintenance food for his animals. The only other ploughing he does is for growing vegetables such as potatoes, carrots and greens for the house.

He grows no corn and very little hay, but uses the grass for silage. He obtains this from between twenty and thirty acres in July and from ten acres in October. There is therefore no harvesting time such as I had known in my young days. Six weeks before the grass is cut the crop is given a dressing of nitrogenous fertiliser. It takes about four or five days to carry the first crop and fill the silage pit. Fermentation is then started by the addition of formic acid. The October crop takes about two days to cut and carry for the second pit.

I was most interested to see the way in which he fed his animals. He had built a new shed with single stalls for two dozen cows and their calves. This he had accomplished with very little outside help. By opening gates the cows could get to the silage to feed; smaller openings allowed the calves to 'creep feed' on their special diet.

He owns sixty cattle altogether and these are all pure Welsh Blacks. Twenty two of these are 'nurse cows' with their calves; there are a few spare heifers and about twenty young beasts (one and a half to two years old) which he is going to sell in the autumn for fattening. Financially he is satisfied that this method of stocking pays, for the price is from twelve to fifteen times that for a similar animal in 1912.

Except in a bad season he buys very little artificial feeding stuff but relies almost entirely on silage.

The two-year olds are wintered in a shed apart from the rest and feed themselves from the silage in the same way.

He has a flock of one hundred and fifty sheep, a hundred are ewes and these he looks after with the help of his well-trained sheep dog. He keeps no pigs, geese or ducks and only a few hens. He feels there is no time to look after them, but they are certainly missed by him and he is seriously considering a pig unit.

He manages all the routine work of the farm by himself with occasional help at the extra busy times.

Many farmers and their wives augment their income by allowing caravan sites to be rented on their land, and by bed and breakfast accommodation, but he feels that his wife's hands are too full to take on extra work and he himself is much too busy. Besides, he had other plans for reconstruction in mind. He has already started on remaking his drive of about four hundred yards with the inevitable cattle grid which has helped farmers throughout the land to keep the animals from wandering.

I came away from Geraint after my last visit thinking that however much his father and grandfather might have objected to the changes they would have been very proud of what had been achieved by one of their own blood stock. I had seen with great pleasure what a young man with common sense, knowledge and, above all, energy and determination could do even in these highly competitive times. What a change from the news and pictures we have been watching of youngsters demonstrating and talking a lot of nonsense about freedom and the perfect world. Here, on the other hand, was an example of what I reckon to be the silent majority of the young generation of today.

There is no limit to what they can and will achieve, and it is as well to remember this.

Looking back to my wonderful holiday in 1912 there was a social aspect to life on the farm which seems to be missing today. Results had been achieved without many labour saving devices. There was enjoyment with every effort until the task was accomplished. Of course there was physical fatigue, anxiety and other natural instincts which were aroused when contemplating the future, but in those days changes were few, the world around appeared very stable and reliable. Today the life is much more lonely, more work is done in a shorter time but there seems to be little time left to look around, to wonder or admire. Are we missing something, or are production and material gain the measure of success in the world today? The old question comes up again — what is the purpose of living?

Modern Medicine — General Practice

The story of medicine is closely bound up with the progress of man in his search for knowledge. It is but natural that he should pay special attention to the health and vigour of his own body. Setbacks, through ill-health for himself and his kith and kin, must have been of great concern to him. In his search, therefore, the human body was of particular interest and had a high priority for his attention.

Scientific medicine did not develop steadily and evenly throughout the years. It did so by leaps and bounds with periods of consolidation in between periods of progress. Clearly we could not expect changes in thought and habits in a free society (whatever that may mean) to be really acceptable by every one all at once.

In olden times infectious diseases came in waves — epidemics — killing and maiming large numbers of people. No one could explain or understand what was happening and very naturally attributed such calamities to outside agencies associated with the supernatural. Gradually, however, as knowledge concerning the body and its diseases improved, so superstition was replaced by a belief in a natural agency whose action could be explained. This newer view was confirmed when Pasteur, during the nineteenth century, discovered the bacillus. We can understand how beliefs that had been 'good enough for my parents and ancestors' were not to be crushed by new-fangled ideas. At first Harvey's explanation of how the blood circulated in the body was looked upon as one such idea. So too was Pasteur's discovery of germs and Darwin's theories of evolution and natural progress. Of course vested interests always fought hard against change and still do today. In this respect at least man does not seem to have changed. We realise that there have always been and always will be eccentric persons within the community who do not follow the accepted views of the majority. We owe a debt of gratitude to a few of these for their ideas and discoveries.

In line with the silent revolution which has taken place in this country during the last thirty years, great changes have taken place in the practice of medicine.

I am grateful to my son Martin for his views and comments on the life of the general practitioner today. His remarks on his practice in a combined rural and urban area in North Wales show how these changes have affected the lives of the people and the work of the doctors themselves.

At the time of the National Health legislation and for the following ten years, doctors have tended to be divided into three main groups, each group working in apparent isolation. These groups were the consultants, the public health administrators, and the general practitioners. The hospital consultants with their virtual monopoly of hospital beds and facilities, the public health section controlling the school health service and health visitors, and the general practitioners dealing with illness in the home and patients visiting his surgery.

Today these three groups of doctors work more closely together. Most general practitioners have access to X-ray and Pathology departments where they can send patients for further investigation. However, more access to hospital beds for the family doctor is to be desired, although some of the new hospitals do have beds available to them for general medical and midwifery cases. Many general practitioners also have part-time appointments as clinical assistants in a hospital, working with and for the consultants. The consultants are realising that much of their present work can be done by medical practitioners allowing themselves to do the work for which they spent many years in training, that is, to consult. There is great benefit to the people of our part of North Wales by the appointment of full-time consultants in all branches of medicine at the Bangor hospitals. This is very different from the state of affairs which existed when we were in practice forty five years ago, when the consultants were part-time specialists and really earned their living by general practice and private consultations. They gave their services free to the voluntary hospitals which are now all state supported. Even in Bristol in 1931 the famous heart specialist, Dr Carey Coombs, told me that he was the only specialist who earned his living as a consultant without private general practice.

The Public Health services too have changed in their outlook and structure. District nurses and health visitors, though still to a large extent employed by the local authority, are attached to the general practitioner to work in his surgery or the local welfare clinic. The liaison between the doctor, nurse and patient is therefore much closer and works for the benefit of all.

There are now fewer single handed general practices than there were when we were in Pwllheli. The doctors have joined together to form group practices, the size of which depend on local requirements, usually three or four in number.

Group practice has come about for a number of reasons, each insufficient by itself to justify grouping, but combined together prove the need for such co-operation, and are of great benefit to the doctors and their patients alike.

By united action suitable premises can be provided from which to work — each member of the group sharing the expense of the building and its running costs. In many areas the local authority provides a Health Centre and the general practitioners rent the building.

The National Health Service has given people the freedom to consult their doctor without fear that they will have to pay a large bill either to the doctor, the hospital or the chemist. This is a wonderful freedom for the patient, but it does put pressure on the doctor who, as a result, sees a large number of patients each day in both the surgery and in their homes. Secretarial help and a receptionist are necessary therefore and can best be provided for a group of doctors working together.

With the improvement in transport and communication facilities and more people owning cars, it is not so important for the doctor's surgery to be near at hand as it was in our practice days.

Last, but not least, the average general practitioner works long hours and under considerable pressure. He would like to be able to lead a normal family life with his wife and children, and by joining in a group is able to take time off-duty and have an occasional holiday. He is no longer the isolated doctor that he used to be, and this is all to the good for both him and the community in which he works.

The proportion of people over the age of sixty five in the population has risen over the last forty years. Although in good health their medical supervision demands more of their doctor's time. This problem is being tackled by co-operation between the doctors and the Social Services enabling them to seek out those who are in need.

The ambulance service of today is both large and efficient. There is no difficulty in obtaining transport for a patient to hospital whether as an emergency or to attend as an outpatient. How different from forty five years ago. From 1925 to 1928 when we were in practice I cannot recollect ever calling on the help of an ambulance. My mind goes back to my early days in Bristol in the 1930's when there was a very poor ambulance service even in that big city. There were only three fully staffed ambulances used by the old Guardians hospital, and three or four used for the transport of infectious diseases. The St John's Ambulance still dealt with accident cases manned by voluntary helpers. I remember submitting a scheme to the City Council in 1930 to raise the salary of the ambulance staff from 22/- a week to 30/- increasing to 34/-, the only condition being that they should be able to drive and hold a St John's Ambulance certificate. The Council approved. This was the skeleton service for a population of 400,000 people. The problem of developing an ambulance service must have been much more difficult and expensive in a scattered population. Now there are ambulance depots all over the country supplied with means of radio communication to their headquarters and to other ambulances, so as to save time and unnecessary mileage, and they are at the call of doctors for accidents or emergencies.

The Health Clinic is now to be found in most towns, and there is one in Pwllheli operating in the house from which we first practised. Here the patients can attend for dental or ophthalmic services as well as other conditions. Infant Welfare and maternal sessions are also held there regularly.

Today's doctor has far more help in obtaining a quick diagnosis of his patient's illness than we did. There is a first class pathology service from the hospital to give quick answers to many types of disease. X-ray test can be carried out not only on sick people but also on apparently healthy patients to see if there is any sign of unsuspected trouble. Other tests that are now carried out include those for cancer of the uterus, X-ray for tuberculosis and other chest disorders, urine testing for early recognition of diabetes, and some infant diseases.

General practice today involves the family doctor in a lot of practical preventive medicine. Excellent vaccines are now available that have markedly reduced the incidence of many infectious diseases such as diphtheria, smallpox, tuberculosis and infantile paralysis. In fact it is probable that many of the younger doctors practising today have never seen a case of diphtheria or smallpox. Measles and whooping cough have become far less serious diseases. Vaccination of babies against smallpox is now not given in many areas because the incidence of complications as a result of the vaccine is now greater than the risk of catching the disease itself. As parents come to realise the facilities and ease with which these injections can be given, more and more children are being immunised against these infections.

Very few babies are born at home, so the general practitioner does not attend many confinements. The mothers are often discharged from hospital after forty eight hours and then the family doctor becomes responsible for her post-natal care. Mothers-to-be are now making good use of the ante-natal clinics and this fact, coupled with the modern treatment now available, has resulted in a lowering of the maternal and infant death rate to a remarkable degree.

The majority of patients do not abuse the Health Service but use it to the full. I am pleased to see all these changes that have taken place in medical practice, but am astonished at the calm way in which this great progress is taken for granted by the present generation. During the last journey of the American astronauts to the moon we watched their achievement with awe and bewilderment, but our younger grand-children were much more interested in the latest adventures of their science fiction heroes on the television screen — they took the moon walk for granted.

Some of the work of a country doctor of today is very similar to that of the general practitioner when we were in practice more than forty years ago. However, much has been radically altered by advances in medical science and changes in governmental social legislature.

Many of these changes have been brought about by improvements in treatment and diagnostic techniques. The discovery of penicillin heralded the start of a complete change in the treatment of many diseases. In the past many of these diseases had very serious outcomes, but today infections like tuberculosis, meningitis, and pneumonia have a very good chance of recovery. Not only are these diseases cured, but now as a result of these new drugs we do not see the chronic disorders such as chronic ear disease, bone infection and rheumatic heart disease that we encountered in the past. Pneumonia is often diagnosed in the first twenty four hours of the onset, and the case improves in a further forty eight hours without the patient being aware of the nature of the illness from which he has been suffering!

I feel I cannot leave this subject without referring to the occasion when the application of the discovery of penicillin was first brought to my notice. It was in the early years of the last World War at a meeting of the Advisory Council of the Nuffield Provincial Hospital Trust of which I was a member. Dr Howard Florey, the Professor of Bacteriology at Oxford University approached the Council to seek assistance for a research project. He was anxious to find a means of preventing the terrible catastrophies that had resulted from gas gangrene in severe wounds of men in the First World War. In his search he had read the paper by Alexander Fleming some years before, which drew attention to the action of a mould that inhibited and even killed the growth of bacteria in the test tube. He wanted to isolate this material if possible and find its composition. He told us that the biochemist, Hubert Chain would join him in his research. We were all most interested and at once recommended all possible support. At the quarterly meeting a few months later I was sitting next to Sir Hugh Cairns, the brain surgeon, and he told me that as a result of Dr Florey's research he had tried the extract he had produced and that became known as penicillin. The cases he had treated were infections within the skull which had responded with quick and remarkable success. As most of his operative work was concerned with such infection he reckoned that as a surgeon he would soon be out of work.

However optimistic we may have been at the time no one was sanguine enough to think that within one generation it would attain such phenomenal results.

Joan had a bad infection of her face whilst serving in the Army and was given a few injections of penicillin. However, in those early days after its discovery the product was not entirely pure and the pain produced by the injection was almost unbearable. She insisted that, following the third one, she would have no more but fortunately the three proved to be sufficient and she made a quick recovery. Since those days the antibiotics have been so purified and improved that they can now be given by mouth.

Like every other new discovery in medicine the antibiotics cannot be administered without careful and measured consideration. Insufficient dosage can produce dangerous results by merely 'wounding' the germs, which then produce offspring resistant to the drugs so creating further trouble. Besides it is possible for a person to become sensitive to these drugs and produce undesirable effects when given them as treatment.

A few years before penicillin was discovered Sulphonomides, chemical compounds, had been given by mouth in cases of bacterial infection. They were found to cure certain types of infection and are still used as alternatives to antibiotics, and are even found to be preferable in some instances. It is worth recording that the research work on these chemicals was carried out at the Middlesex Hospital by Lionel Whitby and were manufactured by the pharmaceutical firm, May and Baker and became known as M. and B. King George the Fifth was one of the early cases to be treated successfully by the sulphonamide drug when he developed a lung infection a year or so before his death in 1936. We had occasion to be thankful for their discovery when our daughter Ann suffered a severe infection of her hand which spread rapidly up the arm. Treatment by sulphonamide cured the infection which might otherwise have resulted in blood poisoning.

The family doctor of today is faced with some problems that we did not have over forty years ago.

There is now a high demand for family planning advice. This has occurred since the introduction of the 'pill'. This form of contraception which now seems remarkably safe has brought much comfort to many parents who wish to plan their family in number and in the length of intervals between pregnancies. There are, however, great social problems when the doctor is faced with the problem of young unmarried girls who request, nay demand, the pill for purely contraceptive purposes. Add to this the fact that nowadays abortions are more freely available and the doctor's predicament is a very real dilemma. He must either supply the pill or arrange an abortion later! Fifty years ago when I was a medical student I remember my teacher, the consultant gynaecologist, stating that pregnancy was the policeman of morality. The policeman has been removed in this modern age of 'permissiveness'.

Another new problem is drug addiction, especially among the younger age group. Not only is this addiction to the soft and hard drugs having a serious effect on the health of these young people, but the greater use of anti-depressants, tranquilisers and sedatives is often replacing the less harmful bottle of medicine we gave to patients forty five years ago. The use of the newer drugs has probably come about because of the increase in the incidence of mental illness in the community. Most of these patients are not ill enough to warrant hospital treatment, but require help and advice from their doctor. Many reasons connected with the modern way of life contribute to this increase in nervous disorders; the rush, the pressures, the unsettled state of the world, the greed of people in the affluent society, and the general lack of a sense of purpose in the life of many people. In spite of all this the majority of folk in this country are healthier than they were when we were young and they have more social security, but are they happier? They should be.

Two human instincts which a doctor frequently meets when attending a seriously ill patient are fear and pain. They must always be taken into consideration both in diagnosis and treatment. These instincts are the same today as they have always been.

Prime Minister Churchill and President Roosevelt in their Atlantic Charter included fear amongst the five freedoms. No doubt that in the midst of a world war they had in mind the threat of wars, and conquests of people, destroying national liberty. No civilised person could disagree with this dictum. History is full of the tragedies of precious lives terminated in fighting for national liberty. On the other hand, from the point of view of the physiologist studying the individual human being, fear is one of the more precious instincts in the process of self preservation. Of course excess fear is always harmful, just as is excess of eating and drinking. But food and drink in moderation are essential for human survival; so too is fear. It is a process whereby the body is alerted to danger — extra sugar enters the blood, the heart is stimulated and the whole body becomes ready for action. I have read much about brave deeds, but never have I read of heroism that had not meant instinctive fear. In fact it may be that because of fear and the alertness produced thereby the hero was able to face the danger and overcome it. My exper-ience has mostly been concerned with sick people and their attitude to pain and death. During the stage of uncertainty and anxiety in an illness the mental strain can be intense and difficult to keep under control. When however, the chances of recovery are known the real character of the person then becomes apparent; despair and confusion, or courage and peace of mind show the true character of the sufferer. I have seen many of both types and my admiration for the latter has been unbounded. In old age the mind has been gradually prepared for life's final stage. Memories of the past or conscience can be calming or disturbing factors in facing the end. I well remember a man who was really frightened of dying because his misdeeds were preying on his mind, and he feared the consequent punishment that would be meted out to him in the life to come. Nature, however, can be kind and frequently there is a state of mental unawareness of approaching death, especially in old age or sudden death.

Some of the cases the doctor sees are sad and touching. I was at the bedside of a young professional colleague who had just returned from hospital where he had been told his illness was incurable. In a matter of fact way he said to me, "I had hoped I would live to finish educating my children, but I shan't." His boy and girl were just entering the University. My own distress and greatest sympathy have been in cases such as this.

Pain, like fear, can be regarded as one of nature's ways of alerting the body to danger. It may be only a signal of a minor ailment, or on the other hand possibly of a more serious trouble, but it cannot be ignored. Once the cause of the pain has been diagnosed and proper steps taken to treat the complaint, it becomes one of the doctor's chief concerns to alleviate the suffering.

Every person reacts in a different way to fear and pain, but from my varied experience in dealing with people I have not agreed with the song, "For men must work and women must weep ..." for I have great admiration for the way in which women face up to hardships and worries in the home. Stability in family life depends so much on the mother, and her attitude to life often reflects on her husband's ability to play his part in the family circle.

The words of the great philosopher, the late President Masaryk of Czechoslovakia seem to be very appropriate in these modern days. He wrote thus:

"Those who assume that health and longevity are secured by well-being and sufficiency and superfluity of nourishment need not be reminded that men do not live by bread alone. Wealth and food are not the only decisive factors. Bodily and mental health are preserved by moderation and morality, and to live healthily a man must have a purpose in life, something to care for, some one to love, and must conquer the fear of death that assails him alike in moments of acute danger and at hours of petty anxiety about health. Civilised man is ever seeking health and happiness yet is unhappy and unhealthy. With all his civilisation he is pitifully lacking in culture."

Few people would disagree with the great Czech leader. However, the Welsh poet has expressed in verse his thoughts about life's struggle and is far from being despondent.

> "O blessedness of living! And how favoured is man
> That he can delight in life within life's span."

(A translation by Sir Thomas Parry Williams of his verse

> "O fendigedigrwydd bywyd! A dyna lwc
> Fod dyn yn cael blas ar fyw cyn chwythu ei blwe.")